I didn't come to teach you.
I came to love you.
Love will teach you.

FREE BONUS
Discover Ancient Healing Secrets That Can Change Your Life

Do you, or someone you love, have a challenge:

- ✓ Physical
- ✓ Mental
- ✓ Emotional
- ✓ Spiritual

Has something afflicted you for years and you want relief?

Our FREE membership website has all the links, videos, and resources from this book, as my gift to you.

You can sign up now at:
www.MyAncientSecrets.com/Belong

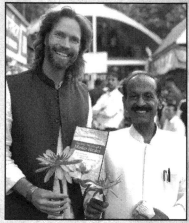

Dr. Clint G. Rogers & Dr. Naram

In Your FREE MEMBERSHIP WEBSITE, You'll Discover:

- ✓ How to instantly reduce anxiety
- ✓ How to lose weight and keep it off
- ✓ How to boost your immunity and energy
- ✓ How to ease joint pain with food
- ✓ How to improve your memory and focus
- ✓ How to discover your life's purpose
- ✓ And much more...

You'll get videos which match up to each chapter, demonstrating the secrets in this book, so you can help yourself and others.

Also, you can experience a powerful game, called *30-Days to Unlocking Your Ancient Secret Power*. As you play, you will discover how to immediately apply the ancient healing secrets in your life. (NOTE: This includes advanced content not found in the book.)

Discover Now at: MyAncientSecrets.com/Belong

Praise for Ancient Secrets of a Master Healer

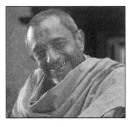

"Dr. Clint G. Rogers has done a great *seva* (service) with this book. The world is in need of great help, as it is polluted not just in the way most think . . . also mental, emotional & spiritual pollution too. The ancient healing secrets in this book are a deeper solution for the world's biggest problems today. I've known and respected Dr. Naram for more than 40 years, personally met his guru master, Baba Ramdas, and know the power of this unbroken lineage ultimately coming from Jivaka (personal physician of Buddha). I've seen Dr. Naram use the ancient healing principles to help the people I've sent to him to reverse and overcome rheumatoid arthritis, epilepsy, severe menstrual bleeding, liver infection, lung infection, multiple sclerosis, heart blocks, cancers, infertility, fibroids, diabetes, thyroid problems, complications in pregnancy, high cholesterol, high blood pressure, hair loss, ascites, urinary tract problems, tailbone fracture, severe hernias, psoriasis, autism, eczema, cervical spondylosis, and brain challenges, just to name a few. Dr. Naram has a *siddhi* (power) for healing given by grace of his master. The secrets of ancient healing revealed in this book are needed more than ever."*

–H. H. Hariprasad Swami (Head of the Yogi Divine Society)

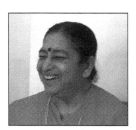

"Dr. Pankaj Naram is a world authority in ancient healing secrets. This book is inspiring, sharing how to infuse these ancient healing secrets into daily life for immense energy, health, and happiness. I am taking his herbs for diabetes and cholesterol and have had extraordinary results. Many Sadhvis in Bhakti Ashram are taking his herbal formulas and have had incredible effects and some completely cured. Whether it be diabetes, thyroid, arthritis, joint pain, back pain, asthma, or more, all are having amazing results. I thank Dr. Clint G. Rogers for this magnificent book, which every human should read."*

–Beloved Premben, Sadhvi Suhrad (Yogi Mahila Kendra)

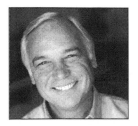

"I know Dr. Naram, who is an amazing being, so when I heard Dr. Clint G. Rogers had written this book about his ancient healing secrets, I got so excited. Most people don't even get 3 minutes with Dr. Naram, but through this book, anyone can be with him on a journey that drops them into his tremendous joy, peace, clarity, and deep wisdom. It's all captured brilliantly in this book as such a phenomenal gift to the world. Do yourself a favor and read this book."*

–Jack Canfield (Success Leader and co-author of *Chicken Soup for the Soul*)

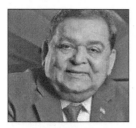

"I have known Dr. Naram for over 30 years and seen his mission to spread healing grow across the world . . . propagating the relevance of ancient healing teachings in modern society. Dr. Naram has brought to the world ancient healing practices that have been lost over the generations. I am sure that you will find this true story, as told by university researcher Dr. Clint G. Rogers, truly fascinating and inspiring, as you discover gems of ancient wisdom that you can apply in your daily life."*

–A.M. Naik (Group Chairman—Larsen & Toubro, one of the most respected CEOs in India & the world)

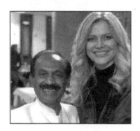

"This book, *Ancient Secrets of a Master Healer*, is like a ray of light for people. I simply fell in love with it. It's so beautifully written and will give a lot of hope to people who need it. I didn't want it to end! I discovered that learning Amrapali's secret is a must. This is definitely one of my favorite books."*

–Arianna Novacco (Miss World Italy, 1994)

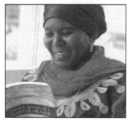

"This powerful book will change so many lives around the world. The Qur'an and Hadith speak about health, with the Prophet Muhammad (peace be upon him) saying: God has not sent any disease without sending a cure for it (Hadith no. 5354). Through the ancient secrets described in this book, so many people will find their cure! I pray more people dedicate their lives to learning and sharing this ancient science to help people throughout Africa and all over the world."*

–Her Excellency Dr. Batilda Salha Burian (Former Tanzanian Ambassador to Japan, Australia, New Zealand, and South Korea)

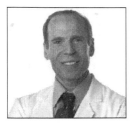

"Remarkable stories of people reversing all kinds of illness and diseases are not 'medical miracles.' These results are predictable when you follow certain principles. Health is your right. Clint is a seeker of truth with a curiosity that has led him on a unique path and mission. He has an impressive knowledge of useful but generally unknown ancient healing techniques. I wish him all the best with this book and in his overall mission to help humanity."*

–Joel Fuhrman, M.D. (President, Nutritional Research Foundation, and 6-time *NY Times* Bestselling Author)

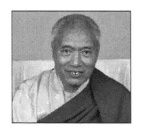

"Wow! This book, *Ancient Secrets of a Master Healer,* is a game-changer for most people's concept of life and health. Each story has such a life-changing impact. As I read each page, I kept thinking about how much I want my son and all the people I love to read this."*

–Wendy Lucero-Schayes (Olympic diver, 9-time national champion)

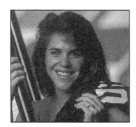

"Following the old traditional healing methods in this book is very good. Dr. Naram is like a great professor in knowing the right methods of making authentic ancient remedies, using real ingredients so it will help others heal deeply without side effects to other illness. Even I had gastric problems, diabetes, and also blood pressure problems. But after having Dr. Naram's treatments for three years, I am much better. It helped me greatly and I feel very well now."*

–His Eminence Namkha Drimed Ranjam Rinpoche (Supreme Head of the Ripa lineage, Nyingma Vajrayana Buddhism)

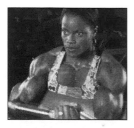

"I'm excited to share these secrets with others and for the wealth of this ancient healing knowledge to spread all over the world, because I know how much it has helped me. I had fibroids and was losing a lot of blood, feeling very anemic. Western doctors wanted my uterus removed, but I believed that if the body creates a problem it can also heal itself. After meeting Dr. Naram, my whole diet changed and I started taking some herbs to help detox and nourish my body. Now I'm pleased to say I enjoy life so much more.

Not only did my fibroids disappear, but also my knees, which had taken a beating with years of professional bodybuilding, got better! It takes faith and changing your mindset from what was to what is. But if you have a burning desire, Dr. Naram can help your dream to become a reality."*

–Yolanda Hughes (2-time winner of Ms. International bodybuilding competition)

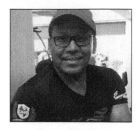

"People call Dr. Naram many things, but I call him my healing guru. For years I've been taking his herbal supplements to naturally support my hormone and testosterone levels, testing my blood reports to see the impact, and I feel great. At age of 73 I'm still in the gym and training for Mr. World competitions. So much is about positive mindset, and I love that Dr. Naram gives me solutions to having great health and accomplishing my dreams in an all-natural, nontoxic way."*

–Sadanand Gogoi (Mr. India Masters, 5-time winner)

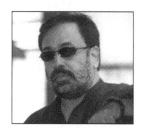

"Once I started reading, I didn't want to put it down! This book brilliantly bridges the East and West, like *Autobiography of a Yogi* did, in a way that is sincere, engaging, and refreshing. This book will spread all over the world, touching millions of lives, as the ancient secrets Dr. Naram shares change our beliefs about health and deeper healing."*

–Pankuj Parashar (Artist, Musician, and Bollywood film director)

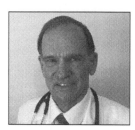

"Every physician trained in Western medicine appreciates its strengths but understands at the same time its limitations. Einstein's thinking forever changed our concept of energy and physics. There is truth to be discovered outside our current thinking and conditioning in medicine as well. Opening our minds to thousands of years of accumulated knowledge in Eastern medicine offers the possibility of complementing and expanding Western medicine with greater effectiveness and healing. This book, *Ancient Secrets of a Master Healer,* has opened my mind and hopefully will yours to a universe where there is so much more for us to continue to learn and benefit from."*

–Bill Graden, M.D.

*Please refer to the medical disclaimer for this book.

More important endorsements for this book can be found at MyAncientSecrets.com

Ancient Secrets of a
Master Healer

Ancient Secrets of a
Master Healer

A Western Skeptic,
An Eastern Master,
And Life's Greatest Secrets

CLINT G. ROGERS, PHD

Wisdom of the World Press

ANCIENT SECRETS OF A MASTER HEALER
A Western Skeptic, an Eastern Master, and Life's Greatest Secrets
by Clint G. Rogers, PhD

Published by Wisdom of the World Press
www.MyAncientSecrets.com

ISBN-13: 978-1-952353-00-0
eISBN: 978-1-952353-01-7

Cover design by Daniel O'Guin
Interior design by Christy Collins, Constellation Book Services

Printed in the United States

Note about new words: This book introduces many words that will likely be new to you—they certainly were to me. For example, when I first heard the word *marmaa* I thought it might be anything—a type of butter, a cuddly animal, or what a drunk pirate might call his mother. (*"Aargh, I luv me dear marmaa!"*) Turns out it is none of these. Some of the words might sound strange at first. I will do my best to translate both their meaning and pronunciation, and, most important, explain how they can apply to you. Each chapter contains notes from the journal I kept of remedies, quotes, and questions. I invite you to be like a researcher with the resources I've shared here. Test them out, and see what happens. There is also a glossary at the back of the book.

*Medical disclaimer: This book is intended for educational purposes only. This book is not meant to be used, nor should it be used, to diagnose or treat any medical or emotional condition. The author does not dispense medical advice or prescribe the use of any technique as a form of treatment for physical, emotional, or medical problems without the advice of a physician, either directly or indirectly. Please find a good physician to consult with on those matters, especially when medications are involved. The intent of the author is only to offer information of a general nature regarding physical, emotional, and spiritual well-being. The cases recorded in this book are remarkable, and it is important to remember that results can vary for each person, depending on many factors, and may not be typical. In the event you use any of the information in this book for yourself, which is your right, the author and the publisher assume no responsibility for your actions. You are responsible for your own actions and their results. Educate yourself fully, so you can make the best choices to align with the results you desire.

Contents

You are not reading these words by accident. You and I are connected, and I believe you were led to this book at this point in time for a specific reason.

Who do you love deeply? And how much would you be willing to help them if and when they desperately needed it?

Love is one of the most powerful forces in you. Never underestimate what it can do.

Even for a science-based university researcher like me, love is the force that propelled me out of my comfort zone to seek solutions that were beyond what I thought was logical or possible.

"Son?" The tone in my father's voice indicated that something was wrong. "Can you come home? I need to talk with you."

It was the spring of 2010. I was a postdoctorate student doing research at the University of Joensuu, Finland, and I received the call while I was traveling in India. I had no idea that the direction of my life was about to change so drastically.

I flew back to the United States as soon as I could and met Dad at his office in Midvale, Utah. As he closed the door behind us, we sat side by side in the chairs in front of his desk. He looked at the floor, not knowing how to start. After what seemed like an unbearably long silence, his eyes slowly moved up to meet my confused gaze.

"I don't know how to tell you this," he said, "but the pain is so intense. At night, I lie awake in so much agony that I honestly don't know if I want to live to see the morning. It's very possible I may not live through this week."

His words took my breath away. I was instantly flooded by sadness and paralyzed by fear. This was not like my father. He was my hero. My rock. By my side in every step of my life. The last time I saw him, he was fine as far as I knew. Sure, he had problems, like everyone who ages. But this? Everything else that seemed important to me, before that moment, faded into the distance as I desperately tried to figure out how to help him.

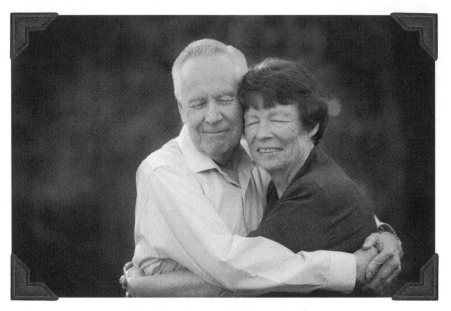

My dad and mom, holding each other.

My dad had already received the best medical care he could find; four distinguished doctors had him on twelve medications for everything from severe arthritis, high blood pressure, and high cholesterol to gastrointestinal and sleeping issues, but the problems were not going away. On the contrary, the pain was only increasing. My mind and body were in shock. I felt like I'd unexpectedly been punched in the gut.

Nothing in my life had prepared me for a moment like this. And nothing I'd done up to that point gave me the knowledge of how to help. For years, I worked helping people invest their retirement savings in the stock market. Financially rewarding, but personally unfulfilling, I went on to get a PhD in Instructional Psychology and Technology. My doctoral studies trained me well for the rigors of academic research, but I knew nothing about healing. As one of my graduate professors once told me, "Accumulating advanced degrees usually just means you know more and more about less and less."

So there we were. My dad said, "Two of my doctors told me this month they don't know what else to do for me." He decided the end was near, and simply wanted me to help him tie up loose ends in case he didn't have much longer. Seeing he'd lost faith that he would recover, I said, "Dad, I never really shared with you what I saw in India. Can I tell you some stories?"

The experiences I shared with him, I share with you in this book. I didn't know if they would help him or not, but I was desperate and didn't know what else to do.

Perhaps that's what life inevitably does to all of us. It brings us to a desperation point, where whatever we have and whoever we are isn't enough. And we know it. It's at that point we either give up or reach for something beyond what we've known—for some greater power.

As I write this, I realize that you—or someone you love—may be at that point now. My prayer is that this book will transform and bless your life by giving you what you need the most: hope and courage. Hope that there are solutions to any and every problem you may face, and courage to keep an open mind to receive them even if they come from unexpected sources.

What happened with my dad helped me understand how love can guide us, even in the darkest times of our lives. I'll come back to that difficult conversation with my dad later in this book, but first I need to share the unexpected series of events which preceded it.

In 2009, I met Dr. Pankaj Naram (pronounced *Pahn-kahj Nah-rahm*) in California. Although relatively unknown in the United States, he was recognized as a master healer by more than a million people in countries across Europe, Africa, and Asia, including India, where he was born. Hailing from a centuries-old unbroken lineage of master healers, which originated with the personal physician for Buddha, each master kept and passed down ancient secrets for helping anyone improve mentally, physically, emotionally, and spiritually.

Personally, I was never attracted to alternative medicine or the people who promoted it, assuming the best medical discoveries would come from well-funded scientific research in universities and hospitals. Those Dr. Naram helped said he instantly knew their problems by just touching their pulse. Then he gave remedies, based on the forces present in nature, that helped them heal, even from "incurable" conditions. Their descriptions made him sound to me like a Jedi healer out of a *Star Wars* movie.

When I met Dr. Naram, I was intensely skeptical. How was it possible to do what I was told he could do? Before the events described in these pages, my attitude about health was what might be labeled as typically American. I consumed a lot of processed and fast food, and whenever I became ill, I would either search Google to find out what I could do, or go to a doctor. For diagnosis of my problem, I expected the doctors to use a thermometer to measure my temperature, poke me with sterile needles to suck blood from my body, and in some cases zap me with electromagnetic radiation or ask me to pee into a small cup. Based on the results, I expected a prescription of a pill or shot to make me better, or in extreme cases, surgery. I assumed they would give me whatever was the best solution according to the latest research. This being the case, I couldn't make sense of how Dr. Naram could so accurately diagnose and effectively help people with what he calls the "six secret keys of deeper healing."

Even after meeting Dr. Naram and seeing the impact his work had on his patients, I had many doubts and struggled to understand what I saw. With the curiosity of a university researcher, mixed with a healthy dose of Western skepticism, I spent time visiting his clinics, questioning Dr. Naram and those he helped. Even writing these words, I realize the story is one I would scarcely believe myself, had I not lived it.

The journey took me from the Lowes Luxury Hotel in Hollywood, California, to the best pizza restaurant in Italy; from the devastation of Ground Zero in New York City to the slums of Mumbai, India; and from my research at the clean and tidy University of Joensuu, Finland, to helicopter rides visiting fire pits and hidden temples in remote areas of the Himalayan mountains. I have now visited, with Dr. Naram, over one hundred cities in twenty-one countries during the last ten years.

Far more amazing than the places were the people, who came by the thousands to see Dr. Naram; from police officers, priests, and mafia to nuns, movie-stars, and prostitutes. I saw women come wearing sarees, burkhas, and bikinis; men wearing work attire or religious robes, and even a couple of naked swamis! Billionaires in well-pressed dark suits came, titans in business, politics, and media; and street kids wearing dirty, crinkled clothes. People brought their children, their neighbors, and their animals. With Dr. Naram, I met powerful saffron-clad rinpoches and lamas in their golden-colored

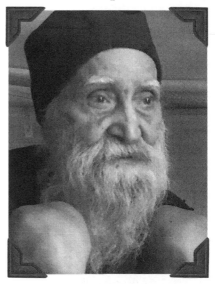

Tyaginath, a 115-year-old Aghori master, whom I met several times with Dr. Naram.

temples; orange-clad yogis or swamis, worshiped by millions, in ashrams by great rivers; and mystical aghori tantric masters cloaked in black, outside burning funeral pyres. I witnessed the problems each faced, and observed how Dr. Naram, dressed in crisp white, helped each and every one.

At clinic locations I recorded videos and documented hundreds of patients' cases, with their permission, taking pictures (some of which appear in this book) and asking to see copies of medical reports and other evidence of their experiences. At least some of their problems (like anxiety, indigestion, high blood pressure, infertility, weight gain, hair loss, and autism) I imagine you will relate to. I often spoke with people before they met Dr. Naram, then again years later, witnessing the entire arc of their transformation.

I also recorded many of my countless conversations with Dr. Naram. They reveal secrets passed down by masters for centuries. To my surprise, I discovered that so many life-changing remedies for our health challenges can be found in our very own homes and kitchens, if we just know what to do.

Fueled by my love for my father, *Ancient Secrets of a Master Healer* traces my journey as a Western skeptic of this ancient healing science to . . . well, you will see as you read. My time with Dr. Naram challenged me and my beliefs about health and life in a way nothing else has. This book captures the first year of that journey. Tragically, Dr. Naram passed away on Feb 19, 2020, only months before the publication of this book. As a result, now this is more important than ever to share.

While sharing these precious secrets with others, I've been shocked how few know that such an ancient science of healing exists. So why were you led to this book? You may not have known deeper healing like this was a choice you had. I'm excited for the way knowing it now can totally change your life and those you love, perhaps showing you more is possible than you ever expected.

Clint G. Rogers, PhD
Mumbai, India
March, 2020

CHAPTER I

Ancient Healing Secrets That Can Save Your Life

The best things in life happen unexpectedly.
The best adventures were never planned as they turned
out to be. Free yourself from expectations. The best
will come when and from whom you least expect it.

–Author Unknown

Mumbai, India

Loving deeply is a force that can lift you to heavenly heights, and sometimes it can put you on a path that leads you into the jaws of hell.

Reshma was praying for any solution to save her only daughter, who was in a life-threatening coma due to complications from blood cancer treatments. "There is no hope," the doctors at the hospital in Mumbai told her. "We've never seen anyone in a condition this severe come out. It's time to let her go." What can you do when someone you deeply love is about to die, and you desperately want to help them but you don't know how? And how would you feel if the things you tried to do to help only made things worse?

Guided by Inspiration or Desperation?

I was in Mumbai, India, visiting the clinic of Dr. Naram, who I'd been told was a world-renowned healer. It was a series of unlikely circumstances that had led me there, which I will share later. For now, I will simply say that being in India was a lot to take in and the activity swirling around Dr. Naram was confusing. On one of my last full days at the clinic, I asked him why people flew in from all over the world just to see him for five minutes. How did they know about him?

Dr. Naram smiled and invited me to the studio to watch while he recorded a TV show on ancient healing which broadcasted in 169 countries. Out of curiosity, I decided to go.

Although Dr. Naram mostly spoke in Hindi during the recordings, the filming process fascinated me. I had never been behind the scenes of a TV show before and was amazed how much painstaking effort went into every detail. It took about forty minutes to

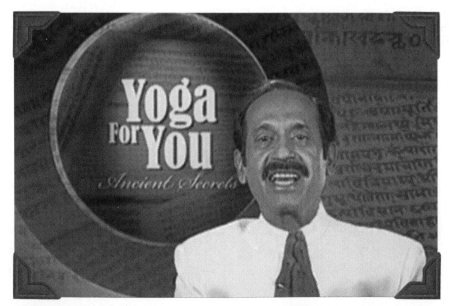

Dr. Naram being recorded for a TV show broadcast by ZeeTV in 169 countries.

get the lighting just right before the director finally said, "Ready, silence, action!"

There was a moment of silence. Then Dr. Naram began speaking to the camera as if to his best friend. Everyone was transfixed by his presence and voice. As it took so long to get to this point, I found myself getting annoyed when I heard a commotion in the room. A woman wearing a green shawl entered the studio, speaking loudly, completely disruptive and utterly oblivious to the silence of the room around her.

The director was irritated as well. But Dr. Naram, on seeing the woman, asked him to stop recording. He walked over and listened patiently as she pleaded, "Dr. Naram, I need you. Please, please, save my daughter's life. She's about to die. I beg you." As she broke into tears, my heart softened.

"I watch your TV show every morning in Bangladesh," she said, "where you help so many people. We use the home remedies you share any time we get sick, and they work. I found the address of this TV studio, got in a taxi, and came here so you can save my daughter."

The woman's name was Reshma. She'd traveled with her eleven-year-old daughter, Rabbat (pronounced *Rah-baht*), over a thousand miles to Mumbai from Bangladesh, to one of the best cancer hospitals in the world. Rabbat had blood cancer, and subsequent to arriving at the hospital she fell victim to a terrible lung infection, one of the unfortunate possible side effects of her treatments. Reshma described how, once smiling and playful, as soon as the infection took hold in Rabbat's body, she quickly slipped into a coma. For eleven days now, Rabbat lay unconscious, 100 percent dependent on a ventilator. Despite having the most expensive medical equipment, top doctors at the hospital were forced to bring Rabbat's chance of survival to almost zero and encouraged Reshma to take her off life support.

Reshma exhausted all of her husband and family's financial resources, going into serious debt, in trying to rescue their daughter. Even if she had the thousand dollars per day it cost to keep her daughter alive in the ICU (Intensive Care Unit)—which

> *"No matter how big the problem or difficulty, never give up hope!"*
>
> –Baba Ramdas
> (Dr. Naram's Master)

she didn't—she was running out of time. The longer Rabbat showed no signs of improvement, the more emphatically doctors urged Reshma to terminate her life support.

Like any devoted mother, Reshma was frantically searching for anything or anyone else who could help. The pressure of removing the life support was mounting when a tiny spark of hope stirred inside as Reshma suddenly remembered Dr. Naram lived in Mumbai. Reshma's desperation and mother's intuition led her to where Dr. Naram was recording, just twelve hours before he would leave the country again. Dr. Naram was traveling so often that he was rarely in India, much less at the recording studio, so Reshma took it as a sign from God.

"You must be here for a reason," Reshma said. "Allah [God] led me to you. You are my only hope!"

That seemed like a lot of pressure to put on someone, and I watched closely as Dr. Naram responded.

He touched Reshma gently on her arm and said, "My master taught me, no matter how big the problem or difficulty, never give up hope!"

Although he was soon leaving the country, he promised to send one of his top students, Dr. Giovanni Brincivalli, to the hospital the next day to see her daughter. Then, turning to me, he said "Clint, why don't you accompany Dr. Giovanni? You might learn something valuable."

I didn't plan to spend one of my last days in India going to a hospital, but I went anyway. That decision ended up being monumental.

The Distance Between Life and Death

The next day Reshma anxiously greeted Dr. Giovanni and me at the entrance of the hospital. She had long dark hair pulled into a tie behind her head and wore a green shawl wrapped around her body. Without wasting time, she quickly walked us to the ICU, where her daughter, Rabbat, lay in a coma. Like intensive care units in other hospitals, it was sterile and melancholic. Four beds crowded this room, each holding someone deep in a coma. A heaviness hung low in the air and I hoped I wouldn't have to stay long. Family members stood by in subdued silence. Their whispers and quietly falling tears penetrated through the incessant beeping of machines and monitors. The bleak atmosphere reminded me of a viewing at a mortuary, and I was struck by the probability that these families, including Reshma's, might soon be standing over a casket or burning funeral pyre that would envelop their loved one.

Dr. Giovanni walked beside Rabbat's bed, dressed in white pants and a white button-down shirt. He had slightly graying, speckled hair and a gentle disposition. As he took Rabbat's pulse, his compassionate eyes, normally accompanied by a broad, cheerful smile, were now dim with concern.

I stood next to Reshma at the foot of her daughter's bed. "Not long ago I watched her as she was playing jump rope, smiling, and eating ice cream in our garden," she told me as we looked at

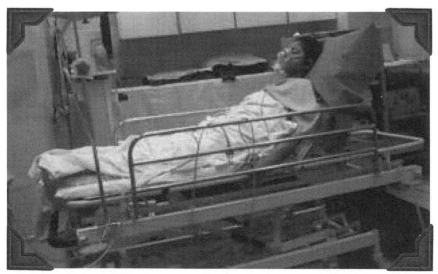

Rabbat, in a coma, photographed by her mother.

her daughter's fragile little body wrapped in a cocoon of blankets. Rabbat was barely breathing. Her eyes twitched while held shut with tiny strips of tape. Her young face and body were swollen and puffy with the lure of death. A sharp needle pierced her wrist and was connected to an IV. The tubes protruding from her nose and mouth helped her breathe, while the electrical wires attached to her chest and head tracked her vital signs.

Unsure of what to say as we stood gazing at her unconscious daughter, I thought of the question Dr. Naram asked me when we first met—the same question he asks everyone. So, I asked it of Reshma, "What do you want?"

"What do you want?"

(Key question
Dr. Naram
asked everyone)

With tears pouring down her cheeks, she looked directly at me, replying in broken English, "All I want is for my little girl to open eyes and say 'Mommy' again." Reshma's voice quivered as she spoke.

The sheer magnitude and ache of her plea pressed heavy on my heart, as I did not know how it could ever become a reality.

Looking around at the high-tech, modern hospital setting, I thought that if anyone could save her daughter, shouldn't it be this place? This medical facility matched any that I'd seen in the United States or Europe. It was one of the best hospitals for cancer treatments, and Rabbat's attending physician was a renowned cancer specialist. As one of the top authorities in his field, not just in India or Asia, but in the world, if he didn't have a solution, it seemed soberingly obvious that there was likely no solution anywhere.

Was it arrogant of Dr. Naram to think his ancient healing methods could defy the odds when the best experts could not? Or maybe Dr. Naram knew there was nothing he could do so he avoided coming and sent his student instead. If so, why couldn't he just be honest with Reshma and tell her he didn't have a solution? Why give her false hope by sending Dr. Giovanni? I worried that Reshma's hopes were misguided, that by putting her faith in Dr. Naram's ancient healing methods, she was setting herself up for inevitable heartbreak.

It was sobering standing next to Reshma looking down help-lessly at her daughter. I began to feel and understand even more the pressure and trauma Reshma was experiencing. She sacrificed everything. She left behind her husband and two young sons in Bangladesh, seeking the best treatment for her only daughter. She was hopeful it was all worth it when Rabbat showed signs of improvement, until that ominous day when a fungal infection suddenly invaded her daughter's entire body. "One day Rabbat started holding her throat," Reshma quietly explained, "saying it felt like someone was choking her. It was shortly after that she went into a coma." The sad reality was that the side effects of the treatments which they'd gone into huge debt for, now threatened Rabbat's life more than the cancer itself. The nurse told Reshma that if the oxygen tubes were removed from her mouth, she would likely survive only a few minutes.

Reshma's love for her daughter was as vast and powerful as the ocean, but was now reaching for the sky and breaking on the sand. Looking down at her daughter, Reshma faced excruciating questions. Was this the end result of all her prayers, money, and tears? Did she have to be the one to make the dreaded choice of ending her daughter's life? How could that be? It was a decision no one should have to face—a mother's unfathomable terror.

Witnessing Reshma's despair triggered emotions that had long been buried inside me. I was eight years old, visiting my own sister at the hospital, not long before her unexpected death. As a boy, I watched my sister suffer and felt helpless to do anything about it. Startled by this memory, as Reshma stood next to me quietly crying, I felt tears swell in my eyes.

In that moment, I was struck by how fragile life is; the distance between life and death for any of us could be only one or two breaths away. I became conscious of the air entering, then exiting my lungs.

Each breath, I understood, is a gift.

My sadness turned into self-conscious discomfort. In that moment I was feeling that perhaps it was a mistake to come to

India at all, especially as I was standing there watching this little girl struggle for each remaining breath, with no idea whether Dr. Naram or his ancient methods would help her.

Perplexed by Reshma's decision to reach out to Dr. Naram—and trying to move beyond my discomfort—I turned my attention to Dr. Giovanni.

Tears & Onions

I watched Dr. Giovanni take Rabbat's pulse and call Dr. Naram to discuss the situation. Dr. Giovanni graduated with a medical degree from the oldest and one of the most respected medical schools in Europe before training with Dr. Naram for over seventeen years. Upon first meeting him, I had wondered why this highly educated doctor from a prestigious medical school would be interested in studying these ancient healing methods at all, much less for such a long time. Despite his background in both Western and Eastern medicine, I questioned how Dr. Giovanni would assess this seemingly dire prognosis.

At the clinic, I saw Dr. Naram or Dr. Giovanni prescribe herbal formulas or home remedies. Although people told me these did help them heal, I suspected it was the placebo effect more than anything else. Perhaps his patients *believed* Dr. Naram could help them and their beliefs created the positive outcome of feeling better. But how could the placebo effect impact Rabbat, who was unconscious? She couldn't just *believe* something would help her and have it be so. Faith is faith, but facts are facts. This girl was in a coma. She couldn't eat anything, making it impossible to swallow home remedies or herbal supplements anyway. How would a natural remedy even be administered?

I listened intently as Dr. Giovanni began to speak. "Dr. Naram says there are things we must do immediately." Instead of suggesting a mix of modern and ancient, Western and Eastern approaches, Dr. Giovanni focused exclusively on the ancient healing methods.

First, he took herbal tablets out of his bag, which he had Reshma crush, mix with *ghee* (a clarified butter, created by cooking all the milk solids out of it), and apply on Rabbat's navel. Dr. Giovanni explained that "in cases where the person cannot eat, this area of the body acts like a second mouth, used in ancient times to help bring needed nutrients into the body."

This approach seemed odd, but since the doctors at the hospital had already done their best and there was nothing to lose, no one was stopping him.

Next, Dr. Giovanni instructed Reshma where and how often to press specific points on her daughter's hand, arm, and head. "According to Dr. Naram's lineage, this deeper healing instrument is called *marmaa shakti*," Dr. Giovanni told Reshma. It was the most peculiar sight watching him, a respected European doctor, engage in these strange activities with so much confidence. And what he did next was utterly bizarre.

"We need an onion," he said, "and some milk." Someone brought him an onion from the kitchen, which he placed on the table next to Rabbat's face. As he sliced it into six pieces, it looked as if the onion fumes caused her eyes to twitch and water a bit. Dr. Giovanni put the pieces in a bowl and placed them on a table to the left of Rabbat's head. Then he had Reshma pour milk into a second bowl and set it on the right side of her daughter's head.

"You must do nothing with the bowls," he explained. "Simply leave them here while Rabbat sleeps."

It was surreal. We were surrounded by the most expensive, state-of-the-art medical equipment, slicing an onion and pouring a bowl of milk. I said nothing, but I thought, *Really?* I didn't participate but watched from the side of the room, not wanting to be associated with such a bizarre, superstitious-looking approach. I couldn't fathom how anything Dr. Giovanni did would make a difference. Reshma, at least, seemed grateful to have something to do besides watching her daughter cling to life.

Since there was no chance Rabbat would be harmed, the hospital staff didn't stop Reshma and Dr. Giovanni, but the looks on their faces mirrored my own doubt that any good would come of it.

When Dr. Giovanni and I left the hospital that afternoon, I didn't think we would see Rabbat again unless we were invited to her funeral. As our driver slowly made his way through the honking horns of a Mumbai traffic jam, a quiet sadness enveloped me. That feeling was all too familiar, a backdrop of my life beyond this day's experience. Memories flooded in. Most people would say I seemed happy and successful from a young age, but deep inside I felt differently. I carried a pervasive melancholic loneliness of which I rarely spoke, even to those closest to me. Instead, I sought distractions from it.

I don't worry about my own death, but the fear of losing someone I love has evoked especially tender emotions in me ever since my sister Denise died when I was a little boy. And what made it even more raw was that, after several attempts, she took her own life.

I remember that night stumbling out from the dark room where I was watching TV, jolted in an instant from the make-believe slapstick world of a sitcom family to my own family's grim reality. I walked towards the living room, confused by the flashing emergency-vehicle lights outside. My dad pulled me into a side room where my other brothers and sisters were huddled together in tears. Through his own tears, he said my sister was gone. She had killed herself.

Even though I was only eight, I asked myself the same questions over and over again. *How come nothing the doctors or my parents did worked? What could I have done to help her? Was there something else I could have said or done to make a difference?* The counselor who met with my family told me I shouldn't feel guilty, but I just couldn't stop.

In the years since, the questions I had as a child morphed into a strong desire to know what life was about. *Why is life worth living? Am I present enough for people I love? Am I spending whatever time I have doing things that really matter? Am I living my life in a way that is worthwhile?*

Being in the hospital with Reshma and Rabbat stirred up all those questions and emotions inside me. Once again, I reflected on how short and precious life really is.

The Unimaginable

The next day Reshma called with astonishing news. Rabbat's dependence on the ventilator had reduced from 100 percent to 50 percent. She was breathing more on her own! Though she remained in a coma and her vital signs were still critical, her condition was stabilizing. Dr. Giovanni seemed hopeful, but I remained doubtful it would be anything more than momentary respite for a mother desperate for signs of hope.

Three days after our visit to the hospital, Reshma called again. "She's awake!"

"What?" asked Dr. Giovanni, surprised.

"She's awake!" Reshma exclaimed. "Rabbat, my little girl, opened her eyes!" With a quivering voice and emphasis on every word, she exclaimed, "She looked into my eyes and called me Mommy!" Reshma's voice gave way to the sound of quiet, grateful weeping. I was shocked. My brain was scrambled. Could this be true?

Dr. Giovanni and I made the drive back to the hospital. He had

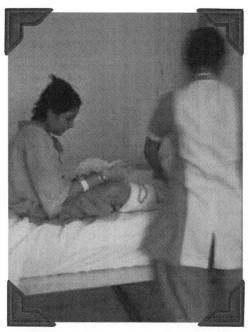

Rabbat being attended to by the nurse shortly after awakening from a coma.

additional herbal tablets for her now that she could swallow. Even as we drove through traffic, I regretfully admit wondering whether Rabbat would still be out of the coma when we arrived. Maybe opening her eyes was a momentary fluke?

My doubts disappeared the moment we walked through the door of her hospital room and saw this beautiful girl, now awake, sitting on the bed!

As Dr. Giovanni took her pulse, Rabbat looked at the many rings on his fingers. Thinking he might be superstitious, she asked him, "Do you have a fear of the future?" We laughed with surprise at how alert and conscious she was. I was impressed by her strong voice, and that she spoke better English than her mother. Her eyes gleamed with life and wonder.

I recorded this meeting with my video camera.

"You look good," I told her.

"Not like before, at home," she said. "If you saw me before, this Rabbat and that Rabbat are not the same."

"Well, you definitely look better than last time I saw you," I said gently.

She smiled.

"How did this begin?" I asked.

Rabbat recounted the story of the pain that started in her body one day and the confusion over why things were getting worse. She shared her last memories before going into a coma, and her first thoughts when coming out. Reshma told Rabbat about who

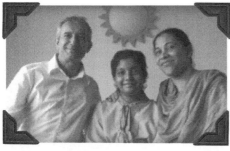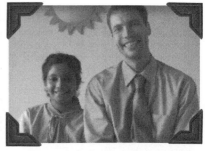

Dr. Giovanni and me with Reshma and Rabbat at the hospital,
after she came out of the coma.

helped her, and so in addition to thanking Dr. Giovanni, she said, "Every thanks in the world to 'Uncle Naram.' He's such a miracle person for saving my life."

"Is Dr. Naram your uncle?" I asked, confused.

She laughed. "No, but in my culture, we call older men 'uncle' and older women 'auntie' as sign of affection and respect."

I smiled at her response, but was thoroughly baffled by what I saw. She'd been in a coma! How could pressing points on her body or placing onion and milk beside her head have helped? Was this result even related to what Dr. Giovanni did, or did she wake up because of some other unrelated factor?

If Rabbat's speedy recovery wasn't already enough to absorb, the most shocking part wasn't *her* recovery alone. It was what we saw happening to the other coma patients who were in the same ICU room.

Contagious Healing

Many people who come through the doors of the ICU do not leave alive. As fate would have it, the sister of the nurse in charge of Rabbat's care was also in a coma in the bed opposite of her. She came to the hospital with a severe liver problem doctors could not cure. As the toxins accumulated in her body, she slipped quickly into unconsciousness.

As in the case of Rabbat, the doctors told the nurse there was no hope for her sister. Seeing Rabbat's remarkable recovery, she asked Reshma what she did to make it happen. Reshma told the nurse, and she proceeded to follow the exact same procedure for her sister.

When we finished visiting with Reshma and Rabbat, the nurse took Dr. Giovanni and me to see her sister. Her eyes, which days before had been closed for what seemed like the last time, were now open and she was fully alert. She smiled the instant she saw us.

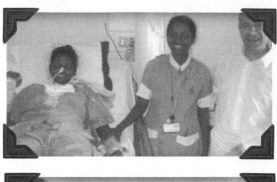

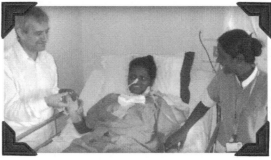

Top: Dr. Giovanni, the nurse, and her sister, the day after she came out of a coma.
Bottom: Dr. Giovanni demonstrating a marmaa point for the nurse and her sister.

"It took some time using the ancient methods," said the nurse. "The changes came slowly at first, until finally, she woke up. And now you can see for yourself the amazing result!" She spoke with elation and gratitude.

The nurse told me that families of other patients began implementing the ancient healing methods, too. Of the four comatose patients in that room, three were conscious and no longer in the ICU, and one had already gone home from the hospital. She spoke of her amazement that these ancient methods facilitated such deep healing, even in cases where the doctors had given up.

I walked out of the hospital in awe, pondering whether people at home in the United States would believe me when I told them what I'd seen. I felt they might think I was smoking something in India! I was glad I had brought my video camera and journal to capture what I'd witnessed.

My Journal Notes

3 Ancient Healing Secrets for Helping Someone in a Coma*

1) Herbal Remedies—Crush required herbs, mix with ghee into a paste, and put on the navel (e.g., the herbal formulas Dr. Giovanni used for Rabbat were tablets Dr. Naram created to support healthy functioning of the brain and lungs*; later, for the nurse's sister, he added one for the liver*).

2) Marmaa Shakti—Here are the marmaa shakti points Dr. Giovanni taught Reshma to press on Rabbat. She pressed this set of points diligently 15–21 times a day, while saying Rabbat's name and loving things to her:

a) On the right hand, at the top portion of the pointer finger, press and release 6 times.

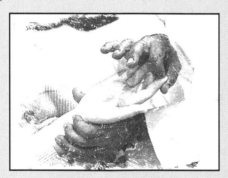

b) On the spot just under the nose and above the top lip, press and release 6 times.

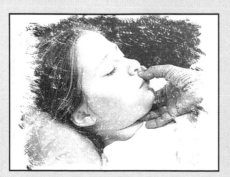

c) Squeeze the head gently 6 times by putting one palm on the forehead, the other palm on the back of the head, curling all the fingers and thumbs to touch and squeeze the scalp.

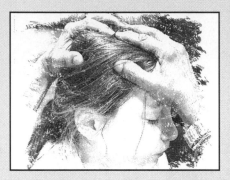

d) In some cases, additional points may be added.

3) Home Remedy—Cut a fresh raw onion into 6 pieces and set in a bowl on the left side of the head; put milk in another bowl and set it on the right side of the head. Leave the bowls there while the person is unconscious.

(Two more secrets for helping someone in a coma are revealed later in this book.)

*Information (including key ingredients) for any herbal formulas and tablets mentioned in this book are listed in a chart in the appendix. Bonus Material: To "meet" Reshma, Rabbat, her nurse, and Dr. Giovanni through the video I captured, and for you to understand this method more deeply, please visit the free membership site (www.MyAncientSecrets.com/Belong).

*Important Medical Disclaimer: This book is intended for educational purposes only. The information found in this book and online is not meant to be used, nor should be used, to diagnose or treat any medical or emotional condition. As of the publication of this book, these ancient secret remedies have not been proven or disproven in any western medical studies that I'm aware of, including clinical trials. They are based on ancient teachings for overall well-being. As you read, please remember the author does not dispense medical advice or prescribe the use of any technique as a form of treatment for medical problems without the advice of a good physician. Please consult with a health care provider for medical treatment. Also, the cases recorded in this book are remarkable, and it is important to remember that results can vary for each person, depending on many factors, and may not be typical. In the event you use any of the information in this book for yourself, which is your right, the author and the publisher assume no responsibility for your actions. You are responsible for your own actions and their results. Educate yourself fully, so you can make the best choices to align with the results you desire.

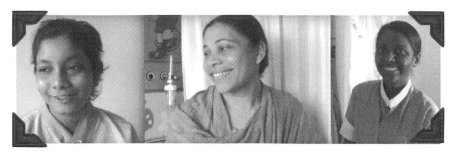

Screenshots from the video I took of Rabbat, her mother Reshma, and the happy nurse.

I wondered, *How did these ancient methods create such profound healing?* If these methods were so effective even in extreme cases of life and death, why didn't more people know about them as an option? What if my family had known of this when my sister needed help? Could it have saved her life? Why onions and milk? How did that even work? Does it work in every case? Where did these "ancient secrets" come from, and how did Dr. Naram learn them? And, above all, why was *I* witnessing this?

It may be helpful now to share how I met Dr. Naram. It was while I was visiting California in October 2009. At the time, I had absolutely no interest in "alternative healing" and no desire to travel to India. I was preoccupied with something much more important to me: trying to impress a girl I'd just met.

Your Journal Notes (from Chapter 1)

To deepen and magnify the benefits you will experience from reading this book, take a few minutes now and answer the following important questions for yourself:

Whom do you love?

_____

_____

_____

_____

_____

What do you want? (For yourself? For those you love?)

_____

_____

_____

_____

_____

What other insights, questions, or realizations came to you as you read this chapter?

_____

_____

_____

_____

_____

CHAPTER 2

95% of People Don't Know
This Important Thing
about Themselves

If you want to make God laugh, tell him about your plans.
–Woody Allen

Los Angeles, California (a few months earlier)

Have you ever met someone who would end up changing your
life completely, only you didn't realize it until much later?

Back in the fall of 2009, I was working in Finland as a university
researcher. During my free time, I was volunteering for an organization based in San Francisco called Wisdom of the World. The project,
called *10 Days to Touch 10 Million*, was working to spread inspirational
messages during the holidays to help decrease depression and suicide. To help capture attention, we created a series of interviews with
famous people that we could promote each day of the event.

One of my roles was to contact and help interview celebrities.
After looking at the list of stars, athletes, and other potential inter-
viewees we'd compiled, my brother Gerald told me that I needed

to meet with Gail Kingsbury. Apparently, she was coordinating an event at an upscale hotel in Hollywood. He said a lot of famous people would be attending, and the only way I could gain access was if I volunteered. So that's what I did.

Dressed in a red, short-sleeve shirt and dark jeans, I felt out of place in the fancy hotel but was instantly comfortable with Gail. She was an efficient event organizer but also a heart-centered person. During a break in our activities, while standing in the hallway, I told her that my primary motivation in volunteering was to meet her and ask her for assistance. Our project touched her, and she said she would help. When I handed her our list of the various movie stars, sports celebrities, and musicians we planned to interview, she looked at it, then paused for a long time. "I'm feeling into the goal of your project, and sensing that most of the people on your list aren't really who you want. Lots are not who they seem to be and they might not match your message," she said, pausing again briefly. "You know who I would suggest?"

"Who?"

"You should really interview Dr. Naram."

"Who is that?"

"He's a master healer from India whose patients included people like Mother Teresa and the Dalai Lama. And today he has a clinic at this same hotel."

A master healer?! That wasn't who we had in mind. I was about to ask her if she'd consider introducing me to anyone else.

Just then Gail's eyes focused on someone behind me. "Amazing. Here he is," she said.

I turned around to see an Indian man in a unique white suit, and a woman with a long, decorative, ethnic-looking jacket walking in our direction. I smiled to myself, thinking that I was not the only one who looked out of place here.

"Dr. Naram, this is Clint," Gail said as they approached us. "Dr. Naram, you need to hear about the project Clint is doing with Wisdom of the World. Maybe you can give an interview, if you have time."

Dr. Naram turned and looked at me. He stood about five feet, one inch tall, a foot shorter than me. He wore a white Nehru-style suit; he had jet-black hair with just a wisp of silver in the front and a clean-cut mustache. He looked young, but what caught my interest were his attentive eyes and his energetic, endearing conversational style.

"Very pleased to meet you," he said warmly. "What is Wisdom of the World?"

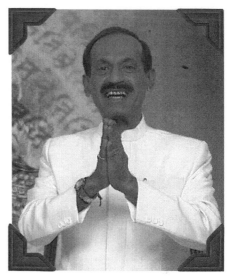

Master Healer Dr. Pankaj Naram.
Photo retrieved from Wikimedia.

I told Dr. Naram about the founder, my friend Gary Malkin, an award-winning musician who has a passion for connecting people with the best things that exist in the world and within themselves. One of Gary's gifts is creating moments of awe and inspiration through music-infused media, to help people remember what matters most. I explained that we were doing a special project for the holidays.

"What do you want?" he asked me. His voice was disarmingly sincere. His inquisitive dark-brown eyes gently focused on my tired and somewhat jaded blue-green ones. My response surprised me.

"I had a sister," I began. "She took her own life. It was one of the most difficult things I've ever faced." This was not something I usually opened up about, and certainly not to someone I'd just met. As I spoke about her I felt the pain of losing her. "I want to do something to help others in the same situation as my sister. I want to help bring more peace to this planet."

"I see. How can I help?" he asked with genuine interest.

"We're doing interviews with remarkable people who might have a message of hope or inspiration. Gail told me that one of the interviews should be with you."

Dr. Naram was leaving the following morning for the next city on his tour, so we arranged to record the interview that night at the hotel after his clinic finished. Having set the time and place, Dr. Naram reached into the pocket of his white jacket and brought something out.

"This is for you, a gift blessed by a great master who is more than 147 years old. You are doing a great work."

His dark hand, adorned with several significant-looking rings, was in stark contrast to the bright-white sleeve of his jacket. In his hand was a shiny ring with an inscription written in what looked like Sanskrit.

With no idea what to make of his claim that someone was 147 years old, I thanked him for the gift. Then Dr. Naram and the woman with him continued down the hall, and I put the ring in my pocket.

After that unusual meeting, I went back to my volunteering duties. While trying to connect with other people we wanted to interview, I reflected on how Los Angeles (LA) was quite a city of contrasts. Whereas television and movies focused on the lifestyles of the rich and famous in Beverly Hills and Hollywood, the fun of Disneyland, and the beautiful beaches of Southern California, I was shocked to discover that there were more than fifty thousand homeless men, women, and children in the city. That's more people than the entire population of Eden Prairie, Minnesota, where I grew up. I got a close-up look into their lives thanks to Les Brown, a well-known motivational speaker who volunteered to help our cause and started our ten-day event by speaking at a homeless shelter in one of the toughest areas of LA.

Throughout the day, my mind returned to the white-clad Dr. Naram. Curious to learn more about who this guy was that I'd be interviewing soon, I went online. There was little information about him in English at that time. I saw pictures of him with some Hollywood and Bollywood stars, like Liv Tyler, famous for her roles in *Lord of the Rings, Armageddon,* and *The Incredible Hulk.* I saw pictures, just as Gail said, of Dr. Naram with the Dalai Lama and St. Mother Teresa. I also found a description of his foundation's work in helping the homeless, sick, and otherwise forgotten.

Other than a tour schedule that showed him visiting many different cities, I found a few articles on random websites about people who had been to India to meet him. They talked about his ability to understand a person by touching the person's pulse. There were a lot of words in the posts I didn't understand, and the whole concept of what he did was strange to me. People claimed that he helped them overcome major illnesses and problems in ways that felt like a stretch of the imagination. Yet it appeared that wherever he went he served the wealthy and destitute alike. And

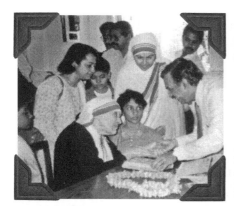
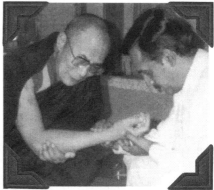

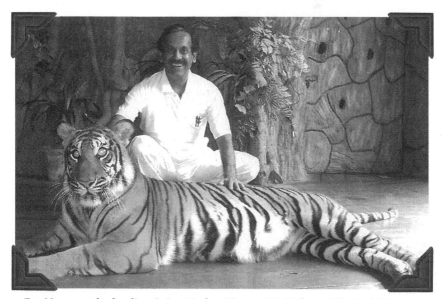

Dr. Naram pulse healing Saint Mother Teresa, His Holiness The Dalai Lama, and a Royal Bengal tiger.

that is what he was doing in Los Angeles, with celebrities from Hollywood and the homeless.

I wondered whether I was doing the right thing by interviewing him. How could any of the stories I read be true? And if what he did was actually effective, wouldn't more people know about him? Wouldn't there be more information about him? From our first meeting, Dr. Naram seemed sincere, likable, and approachable. I enjoyed his alertness and openness. Still, I wondered: *Was this just some kind of an act?*

My training as a university researcher dictated that I investigate further, until I could prove things one way or another. With that in mind, I headed to the hotel room that served as the lounge area for Dr. Naram's clinic.

There were still a few people waiting to be seen by him, so I sat and waited. On the table I saw the same pictures I'd seen online. When it was finally my turn to go in, Dr. Naram greeted me with a smile.

A 125-Year-Old Master?

I wondered whether Dr. Naram would be low on energy by the end of his clinic. Instead, he was brimming with life and so completely present with me, it took me aback. With my video camera on, I asked Dr. Naram to introduce himself.

"I had a master who lived to be 125, who had a master who lived to be 145, in an unbroken healing lineage of masters that goes back more than 2,500 years. This lineage is called *Siddha-Veda*. In the lineage still alive today is my master's brother, who is the one that blessed the ring I gave you. He is now 147 years old. Each master lived to more than 125 years, knowing and passing down secrets to long life, health, and happiness."

I had no idea how to respond. If it were true people lived that long, wouldn't it be widely known? Wouldn't the people he mentioned be in the *Guinness Book of World Records*?

"The first master in our lineage was Jivaka. He was the personal physician for Lord Buddha. You can imagine how enlightened a healer must be to work that closely with Buddha. Jivaka's other famous patients included Amrapali, considered to be one of the most beautiful women in the world, and the Indian King Bimbisāra. Jivaka and each of the great masters of this lineage recorded in ancient manuscripts the secret knowledge about achieving vibrant health, unlimited energy, and peace of mind at any age."

Everything Dr. Naram said was filled with earnest enthusiasm.

"When I first met my master, he was around 115 years old, or he would say he was 115 years young, with many years to go. And at this great age, he was still helping sixty to eighty people every day who came to him with their health challenges."

When I asked Dr. Naram how someone could live so long and still be working, he gave me a "secret recipe" from his 125-year-old master for unlimited energy. It involved soaking fennel, almonds, and dates overnight and mixing them together in the morning. I doubted I would ever use it, but I wrote it in my notebook anyway.

"Thank you," I said. "But how are you doing things other people think are impossible, like healing from seemingly incurable conditions?"

"It's not me, but the ancient secrets of my lineage. I give credit to my master. Do you know the term 'conveyer belt'?"

I nodded.

"I am like a conveyer belt, delivering the ancient secrets to the modern world. And although what happens often looks like magic, it is really an ancient science; it is a technology of transformation for deeper healing."

Right, I thought to myself.

Finding Seeds of Hope

Returning to my initial reasons for doing the interview, I asked him, "What do you think can help people who struggle with loneliness, depression, and even suicidal thoughts during the holidays?"

"Very good question," Dr. Naram answered. "I have seen depression and suicide impact very famous beloved stars and those who are unknown, both poor and super-wealthy people. I've known atheists and even spiritual leaders with millions of followers who committed suicide. Anyone is at risk to lose someone they love this way."

Dr. Naram shared how he was contacted regularly by those who were depressed and suicidal, and that he was eternally grateful each time he felt the blessing of his master in knowing how to help them. "Most important thing is to understand them, not to judge them. Some kids attempt suicide just to get the attention of their parents, begging them to understand their pain and frustration. Once the parent understands, things can get better. Those struggling with depression face a big challenge. And my master taught me how to help anyone come out of it as a winner."

I listened carefully.

"Most people don't know what it's like to be so depressed that you want to kill yourself," Dr. Naram continued. "What makes it so someone wants to hurt themselves? Some reasons include not being able to face fears, frustrations, heartbreak, guilt, anger, loneliness, or financial problems. Each of these can almost paralyze the brain. My master said there are eight different kinds of fears people may face. One of the most powerful challenges on this planet is the fear of rejection. Once a boy or girl, woman or man, feels rejection and heartbreak from a parent or a love partner, their mind may spin into depression. And can you imagine what a homosexual boy or girl in some countries must feel if they face rejection by their society, or even by God? It is actually impossible for God to reject them, because God is in them and God is love; but that is how they can feel, rejected by everyone, and it hurts. It's a very serious issue.

"Then some people have chemical imbalances in their brain, bipolar conditions, manic depression, or struggle from side effects of drug and alcohol abuse. Fear from so many sources can paralyze the brain to not see possibilities of how to get out. My master taught me the secrets of how to help people get out of any of these challenges."

Dr. Naram told me a story of a father and daughter who called him from Rome. She was in love, a euphoric kind of love. Then she and her boyfriend broke up, and she spiraled into severe depression. She said, "Dr. Naram, I lost myself, and now I hate myself. There's a sharp pain in my heart. I stopped living and started dying. I can't take any responsibility. Life feels impossible, and I'm always putting myself down. If someone appreciates me, I feel they are false speaking."

The girl lost her job, could not sleep at night, broke out into sweats, and was overwhelmed with anxiety. Physical pain felt better than emotional pain to her, so she hurt herself. She was taken to a psychiatric hospital and given drugs that made her feel empty, unable to focus, as if her brain was in atrophy. She said, "I feel no joy, no pleasure, and nothing interests me anymore."

The girl's father was tormented by the pressing concern that each morning he woke might be the day that she would succeed at killing herself. He told Dr. Naram he felt constant guilt and wanted to help, but everything he said or did seemed to hurt her more. All he could do was hold on to hope that one day things would improve.

Dr. Naram told me, "I asked the girl, 'What do you want?' And she said, 'I want people to understand me and not judge me! Deep down I'm unhappy. In my heart I feel sad and angry at my disease. I'm afraid that I can't help myself. I want to know how to rebuild my life, let go of the past, and move forward. I want to be in life again, happy. And I want to discover and understand the meaning of existence. But I need help!"

Dr. Naram's story made me think of my sister and the times I visited her in the hospital. I had no idea the kind of heartbreak that led her to depression.

"So how do you help anyone feeling like this?" I asked.

Dr. Naram responded by sharing another story. There was a man in a rocky marriage. His wife threatened three times to divorce him, and each time Dr. Naram helped them discover what they really wanted and to work through their differences. The problem this time was more severe than ever. This man lost over a hundred million dollars of other people's money in a couple of days during a stock market crash. Some of the money came from friends and from his wife's parents. His wife's father had given him their entire savings for retirement. The investments were growing and everyone was happy until the crash; now he didn't know how to face them.

Late one night his wife called Dr. Naram in a panic. As her baby cried uncontrollably in the background, she said, "My husband is sitting right now on the ground in front of me. He has a gun in his mouth, his finger on the trigger!"

Dr. Naram said, "Can you put the phone next to your husband, on speakerphone? And then can you walk out of the room, so I can speak with your husband alone?" She did so.

Dr. Naram said, "Namaste," and then said his name. "What do you want?"

He pulled the gun out of his mouth long enough to say, "I want to end my life."

"Very well," Dr. Naram replied. "How can I help you to die?" There was a long pause. The man was shocked. "I want to help you achieve what you want. If you want to die, then how can I help you?"

"Don't joke with me, Dr. Naram."

"What is it you *really* want?" Dr. Naram asked him.

Dr. Naram explained to me that the questions he asked were part of the method taught by his master to help people overcome suicidal thoughts, but that he didn't recommend others do it without proper training. As Dr. Naram spoke with this man, he discovered that what he truly wanted was to know how to get out of the situation he was in. He wanted to hope that things could get better, and for the pain to go away.

Dr. Naram asked him to put the gun down so he could press a marmaa point to help him accomplish what he wanted, and immediately the man felt calmer. Next, Dr. Naram instructed him to mix some ingredients from his kitchen as part of a home remedy (½ tsp. ghee with a thread of saffron and a pinch of nutmeg, warming it slightly and putting two drops in each nostril). This made him feel even calmer, which, in turn, allowed him to regain perspective.

"It was not a quick fix," Dr. Naram continued. "It took time. But this man committed to doing what was necessary for deeper healing. He changed his diet to eat foods that would nourish good thoughts and emotions. He took home remedies regularly, like mixing some ingredients together with ghee and taking them twice a day. The masters in my healing lineage also created certain herbal formulations that help nourish and rejuvenate the parts of the brain and body, which have been exhausted, so people can connect again with the happiness and purpose inside of them. Again, it's not a quick fix, but it works when people commit to the process. I also gave him other marmaa points which helped stimulate his creativity, too. His creative power came back so much, I'm proud to say, within a couple of years, he earned back everything he lost, and more. He paid back his father-in-law and all his friends with interest."

Dr. Naram emphasized, "My master taught me: 'Every adversity—every difficult situation or heartbreak—has within it the seeds of equal or greater benefit.'

"But first, all of us need to discover: Who am I?" Dr. Naram continued. "In life, most of our challenges come when there is a block or an imbalance or both. We need to discover what the block is and where the imbalance is. Imbalance can be *vata, pitta, kapha,* or a combination." I didn't recognize these terms, but before I could ask for clarification he continued. "Once you know who you are, what your blocks and imbalances are, then you can know what food is your medicine. We need to pay more attention not only to food we are giving our body, but also to the thoughts we are feeding our mind with, and the attitudes we feed to our emotions. Ancient secrets provide guidance on each."

I listened, not believing what Dr. Naram said could be true. My sister was on heavy medications for suicidal depression and that didn't even help. How could pressing certain points on the body and making dietary changes create this kind of impact at such a critical moment in someone's life? What Dr. Naram proposed seemed too simple to be true.

"What happened with the girl?" I asked.

"Aha, yes! She is a perfect example. Since Dr. Giovanni was in Rome, I asked her to see

> *"Every adversity—every difficult situation or heartbreak—has within it the seeds of equal or greater benefit."*
>
> –Baba Ramdas
> (Dr. Naram's Master)

him every four days, for him to perform a specific marmaa on her, helping her get very clear on what she wanted, and cleansing out the old garbage in her system. She felt a little better quickly, and in two months found a new boyfriend whom she wanted to marry. But that was simply out of revenge to her first boyfriend, and so the relationship fell apart and she had a setback in her progress. I told her, 'We need to build you up so you are not having a relationship just to avoid emptiness and pain.' Then she became really committed to her future. I gave her some home remedies and herbal supplements that she took regularly, and she made a big change in her diet. I taught her which foods to avoid that invite negative emotions, and which foods to eat which can foster positive emotions.

"God is within each of us, and we all have a purpose to discover."

–Baba Ramdas
(Dr. Naram's Master)

"Again, it took time, it was not a quick fix, but she began to have more confidence in herself. And after we worked with her for two years, she was so full of confidence she could face any kind of rejection or challenge and it wouldn't affect her. She discovered her dream was to be a teacher and she got a job at a school where she became a great one. Not long after, she met a man whom she fell deeply in love with, more than with anyone before, because she also loved herself. It has been almost nine years now, and she has two kids. With both of her kids she does certain marmaas and feeds them specific foods so that they grow up with healthy emotions and confidence in themselves."

"What advice would you give for anyone who is feeling sad or depressed now?" I asked.

"The most important thing to know for anyone is who you are, where you are going, and what can help you to get there," Dr. Naram continued. "My master taught me that God is within each of us, and we all have a purpose to discover. But you can't see or feel that when you are depressed. One way to begin to come out is by doing the same things I gave to that man and that girl."

My Journal Notes

Three Ancient Healing Secrets to Help Calm Your Mind, Re-Balance Your Perspective, and Stimulate Positive Emotions: *

1) Marmaa Shakti—Every day, have a daily discipline to do this 6–9 times a day. Put your left hand on the back of your head for support, and with your right hand, press and release the marmaa shakti point just under the nose and above the top lip, 6 times. Each time you press the point, take a deep breath. You can do this for someone else or just on yourself.

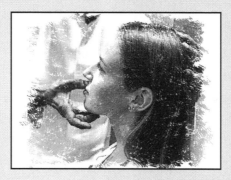

2) Home Remedy—Mix the following ingredients: 1/2 tsp. Ghee, 1 pinch nutmeg, and 1 thread of saffron. Slightly warm the mixture, tilt your head back, and put two drops in each nostril. Do this 2 times a day.

3) Home Remedy—Mix and eat the following ingredients:
  Brahmi churna powder 1/4 tsp.
  Jatamasi powder 1/8 tsp.
  Turmeric powder 1/2 tsp.
  Ghee 1 tsp.

Mix the above ingredients into a paste, and take twice a day (first thing in the morning, and before food in the evening).

*Bonus Material: To see a demonstration of pressing the marmaa shakti points and to discover more secrets which can help in this area (e.g., suggestions on which foods you can eat to promote positive emotions), please refer to the videos in the free membership site, MyAncientSecrets.com

Meeting God?

"What do you mean by 'God is within each of us?'" I asked.

"In India we have a concept for when an unexpected guest comes to visit your home. It is called 'Atithi Devo Bhava'—which means you treat any guest, whoever it is and as inconvenient as their visit may be, as if God himself has come to visit your home. In my healing lineage of Siddha-Veda we take that very much to heart."

"So you believe anytime you meet someone, you are meeting God?" I asked.

"In India we greet people by saying *Namaste* (pronounced *Nah-mah-stay*) or *Namaskar* (pronounced *Nah-mah-skar*) and pressing our hands together in front of our hearts. This greeting means 'the divine God/Goddess in me bows to the divine God/Goddess in you, and I honor that place where you and I are one.'"

"So is Siddha-Veda a religion?" I asked

"Siddha-Veda can help people spiritually, physically, mentally, and emotionally, but it is not a religion. It is a school of thought that anyone can benefit from. These ancient healing secrets are beyond religion, beyond politics, race, caste or creed. They work for everyone universally—just like a car can get you where you need to go regardless of your religion, the color of your skin, or your sexual orientation. Those in my lineage are super-specialists, trained by a line of great masters in the ancient secrets to help anyone who is experiencing pain or dis-ease in body, mind, or emotions to release it. When a person comes to us seeking help, we see the God in them. We do not feel we are obliging them, but that they are giving us a gift. We are honored they came to us. My master taught me that my duty as a healer is simply to help clean the temple to make the God in them happy.

"Consider the cases of those in severe depression, even to the point of feeling suicidal. They are not those heavy feelings of sadness, fear, or anger. That is not who they are. But their minds and bodies are conditioned in such a way that they do not realize this. They feel those emotions and don't know how to let them go. They fear that their problem is so big there is no escape. In that state, you cannot see a happy future at all. So how do we help those who feel sad, mad, or afraid? How do we help clean the temple of their bodies, minds, and emotions so the God in them is happy? This is what my master taught me."

I didn't know what he meant by that, but before Dr. Naram could explain, it was time to end the interview. I had far more questions now than when we had begun.

An Ancient Technology

As I packed my camera, Dr. Naram asked, "What is your work? What exactly do you do for a living, Clint?"

"I'm volunteering on this project with Wisdom of the World because I believe in it," I said. "But I work at the University of Joensuu in Finland as a postdoctorate researcher." I launched into the usual explanation of my work. "I teach about computers, culture, technology, and innovation. My personal interest is how innovation in technology can be used creatively to decrease poverty and increase peace-building."

Dr. Naram was intrigued. "If you are interested in peace," he said, "I need to introduce some people to you."

He reached into his pocket and pulled out an old Nokia phone handset with a small LCD screen. "Since you know about computers, can you show me how this works? People talk about their 'Blackberries,' their 'Apples,' and I get so confused thinking they must mean food, but no—it is their phone! They say this one I have isn't a smartphone. Is it a dumb phone?"

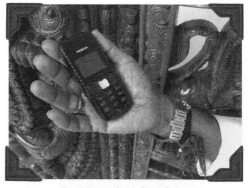

Dr. Naram's Nokia phone.

"Ninety-five percent of people on this planet do not know what they want."

–Dr. Naram

I smiled. His question was endearing and humorous. He wanted to know how to save new phone numbers and how to read and send text messages. While I taught him step by step what to do, he watched with the anticipation and awe of a child. When he successfully saved my number into his phone, he said with triumphant joy, "Aha—I did it! This is an amazing machine, huh?"

Recalling something he said earlier, I asked him, "You mentioned that your master gave you technology, or tools. Technology or tools to do what? What do you mean?"

"Good question. Believe it or not, my master taught me a billion-dollar secret. He said that 95 percent of people on this planet do not know what they want. They just don't know what they want! So, they spend most of their lives window-shopping. Trying out this thing or that thing, this job or that job, this spouse and then another spouse, but are never fulfilled.

"My master said 3 percent of people on this planet know what they want but never achieve it. They don't have the right tools. One percent know what they want, and they achieve it, but these achievers can't enjoy it. In the process of achieving, they get high blood pressure, high cholesterol, back problems, family problems, relationship problems, and what not. Ninety-nine percent of all people fall into those first three categories. Only the remaining 1 percent of people know what they want, achieve it, and then enjoy it."

Hearing these numbers, I wondered: *Am I part of the 95 percent that don't know what they want? I have a lot to be grateful for, so why am I still unsatisfied much of the time? Is my life headed in the right direction?*

Dr. Naram continued, "The ancient healing system of *Ayurveda* that can be learned at universities in India is known as 'the science of life.' The *Siddha-Veda* (or *Siddha-Raharshayam*) of my lineage goes a step beyond that. Siddha-Veda contains the secrets for deeper healing. The ancient secrets of my lineage can only be learned directly from a master to a student, as a super-specialty, a technology of deeper healing. Part of Siddha-Veda's healing secrets or technology helps people *discover* and then *achieve* what they want, and in a way that they can then enjoy what they have achieved."

He paused and said to me, "The technology I don't understand, however, is the one that they call *internets*."

I laughed that he pronounced it with an "s" at the end.

"Tell me," he said. "Do you think the internets could help me reach more people? Physically, I can't meet with more per day than I already do." Turned out he saw about a hundred people a day in Europe, the United States, and Australia, and three hundred a day in India. And I couldn't imagine how that was even possible.

"I know you could reach more people with the *Internet*," I said, emphasizing the correction. "But, honestly, I still don't understand exactly what it is you are doing." I liked being with him, it felt good. He had a youthful innocence and playfulness, combined with a depth of care that was refreshing. Only I didn't know how I could help him, especially when I didn't understand a lot of what he was talking about.

Dr. Naram said something I did not expect: "Why don't you come to India and see for yourself? There are some people I want you to meet."

Surprised and confused by the invitation, I didn't respond.

"Some things may not make sense to your brain at first, Clint," Dr. Naram continued, "because you are coming at life looking through a different lens. You can't understand what I am doing, but being around it, you will start to feel a molecule of hope inside you, and you will be happy. You might not exactly know why at first, but slowly, slowly, things may become clearer to you."

Though touched by his invitation, I found it hard to take it seriously and had no intention of going to India any time soon. So I changed the topic to something that intrigued me.

"How do you understand someone by just touching their pulse?"

"Would you like to experience it?"

I nodded, and he asked me to hold out my hand. He placed three fingers on my wrist and closed his eyes before speaking.

"Do you get headaches sometimes? Sometimes stomach problems? There is an imbalance of *pitta*, and some *aam*, which are toxins. But otherwise you are very healthy."

Although what he said about my headaches and digestion was accurate, I was more confused than impressed.

"I don't understand. What is *pitta*?"

"Fire," he said, "or the element of fire in your body. It is out of balance a little, but don't worry, we can help." He jotted down the names of several herbs unfamiliar to me on a sheet of paper.

I couldn't help but wonder if his trick was to tell people something was off, using concepts they didn't understand, just so he could recommend a product they needed to buy in order to fix the supposed "problem."

I imagined myself talking to someone, making up a problem and saying, "Oh no, not good. You have a serious beep-bop-boop imbalance, very unfortunate. But don't worry, you are in luck, because I have the magical beep-bop-boop cure here in tablet form for one low price of only one hundred dollars."

That's how I felt when Dr. Naram told me I had a "pitta imbalance." I thanked him for the interview and said goodnight.

That Awkward Moment

After leaving the room I gave the sheet of paper with the names of the herbs to Marianjii, who was with Dr. Naram when I first met him in the hallway. She shared more about the herbs and diet recommended, and took people's payment. She explained the *doshas*, or elemental types, and how certain elements in the body become imbalanced and create problems. "*Pitta* is the fire dosha," she said. "*Vata*, the wind dosha; and *kapha* aligns with water/earth. An imbalance of the doshas leads to problems that are predictable and resolvable. Feeling someone's pulse helps Dr. Naram and master healers like him to identify imbalances and blocks in anyone's body." Marianjii then asked me, "What kinds of foods do you eat?"

I described the microwavable burritos, pizzas, and other foods that were easy for a single, postgraduate researcher to eat. She scolded me and told me to take better care of myself. She described the four herbal supplements that Dr. Naram suggested to rebalance my constitution and remove the *aam* (pronounced *ahhm*; sometimes called *ama*), or toxins, from my body.

That's when I started to get antsy, waiting for what I suspected was coming—the awkward moment when she would ask me to buy the herbs and I would say no. But that moment never came.

"In honor of the work you are doing," she said, "we are gifting you two months' worth of herbs."

Surprised, I thanked her. I left with no idea what to make of one of the strangest meetings I ever had.

One week later, the herbs arrived at my home. I took them for a few days, out of curiosity. Part of me wondered whether I would suddenly notice a miraculous result, but instead I had a slight stomachache. *What if rather than helping me, they were harming me?* I didn't know and had no idea who to ask, so I put them, along with the ring he gave me, in a drawer that I rarely opened. As I returned to my day-to-day life, Dr. Naram faded from my mind.

The Power of a Woman

I might never have given Dr. Naram and his "magic" herbs another thought, but then something changed.

A couple of weeks later, I traveled to California again. This time I went with one of my best friends, Joey, to San Diego to promote the project we were working on. One day, as we sat in a juice café near the beach, he introduced me to a woman named Alicia.

Remember I said, at the end of the last chapter, this began with a girl I wanted to impress? Alicia was that girl.

She was gorgeous, with sparkling blue eyes, thick brown hair, and a fair complexion. She had on the sort of colorful, loose-fitting clothing you'd wear to a café near a beach in San Diego. Her voice and attitude were playful yet sincere. And early on in the conversation I felt her innate spiritual sensitivity, which I found myself drawn to.

Wanting to know more about her, I started doing one of the things I do best when I feel awkward: ask questions. Alicia told me about her passion for something called *Ayurveda**. She described it as an ancient Eastern healing system that looks at a person more holistically than Western medicine does.

"The word 'Ayurveda' can be translated as 'the science of life,'" she said.

Science of life, I thought. *What's that?* Although Dr. Naram shared that definition with me, and it sounded funny then also, somehow I was much more interested when it was coming from Alicia.

Though skeptical of the whole topic, I was interested in science—and I was *very* interested in her.

"You know," I said, "I recently interviewed a guy who's supposed to be a 'master healer' from an ancient Himalayan lineage that he called *Siddha-Veda**. He was a doctor for Mother Teresa, the Dalai Lama, Nelson Mandela, and thousands of 9/11 firefighters."

I was grasping for anything related to her interest in order to keep the conversation going. And why not do some name-dropping too, in case it made her interested in me, right?

I've never been good with women. One time I dated a girl who told me she had to pray to be attracted to me. True story. I guess I was just more comfortable behind a computer or writing an academic research paper than trying to understand the mind of a woman. But even I could tell that something in this conversation

---

*For a chart comparing similarities and differences of Siddha-Veda, Ayurveda, and modern medicine, see the appendix at the end of this book.

with Alicia was working. She looked excited about what I said, so in my awkward attempt to connect more with her, I offered to introduce her to Dr. Naram.

"You could do that?" she said. "That would be a dream come true!"

To my shock, this stunningly beautiful woman smiled at me, wrote down her phone number, and asked me to stay in touch!

The bliss I felt turned quickly to anxiousness, as I wondered whether I could actually deliver on what I'd offered her. Now feeling pressure, I called Dr. Naram's office in Mumbai to find out if his invitation to come to India still stood.

I had no idea that what began as an attempt to impress a beautiful woman at a California beach-side café would lead me on a trip to India with her, just a few months later, headed to the clinic of Dr. Naram.

Your Journal Notes

To deepen and magnify the benefits you will experience from reading this book, take a few minutes now and answer the following important questions for yourself:

On a scale of 1–10 (1 being very low, and 10 very high), how happy are you in your life right now? And what are the things that you can think of that make you happy?

_____

_____

_____

_____

Dr. Naram's master said, "Every adversity—every difficult situation or heartbreak—has within it the seeds of equal or greater benefit." When was a time in your life where you saw a hidden benefit come from a challenge you have faced?

_____

_____

_____

_____

What other insights, questions, or realizations came to you as you read this chapter?

_____

_____

_____

_____

CHAPTER 3

Mystical India, an Ancient Science, and a Master Healer

Miracles happen every day. Change your perception of what a miracle is and you'll see them all around you.

–Jon Bon Jovi

Mumbai, India

My first visit to India was eye-opening. The sights, sounds, smells, and flavors left an indelible impression.

Huge skyscrapers and apartment buildings were surrounded by modest hand-made structures that housed a startling number of people. Various aromas from street food vendors mingled with exhaust from vehicles. People in Western clothes mixed with those dressed in traditional Indian attire: women in beautiful saris and the occasional bearded or bald man wearing only a loosely wrapped orange robe and sandals.

Mumbai's bustling streets filled with streams of people and vehicles of all shapes, sizes, and colors. I came from such a different world. Growing up in Eden Prairie, Minnesota, I was used to wide-open fields and mostly empty streets. In most places in the United

States, honking is rare. When you do, it means someone is usually angry or scared. In Finland, where I was living at the time, honking was even more unusual. In India, by contrast, drivers honk nonstop. They're not angry, though. They are gently yet persistently saying, "Hey there, I'm here, trying to get through."

I saw huge cows, considered holy in India, roaming freely like queens anywhere they pleased—on sidewalks, at intersections, even in the middle of the busiest streets, obstructing traffic flow. Quite often those holy cows also deposited their holy sh** on the sidewalk, and no one seemed to mind.

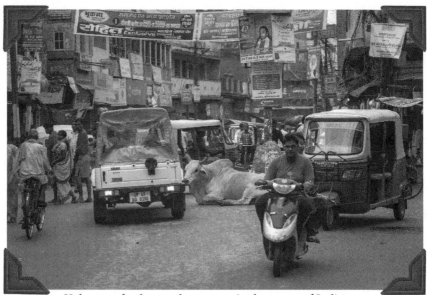

Holy cows freely wander, or rest, in the streets of India.
Photo retrieved from Alamy.

Surprisingly, people don't get frustrated or angered when a car (or cow) cuts them off, or if the ride takes an hour longer than expected. Everyone takes traffic in stride, unlike in America, where they seem to take it in strife. On the back of colorfully decorated trucks or rickshaws, I saw a string tied with green chilies and lemons for protection. Was this their version of a lucky rabbit's foot? It was funny seeing hand-painted signs on the back of most trucks saying *Horn OK Please.* I guess it encourages smaller vehicles to let truck drivers know they are trying to get through.

Walking the streets of Mumbai, with people and cars moving in every direction, I marveled at how more people don't get injured or killed in all the chaos. *Maybe that's why they're all interested in developing their "third-eye."*

Speaking of which, as one of the oldest continuous civilizations, where the written word originated and where Gandhi was born, India has an interesting spiritual ecosystem and culture of inner development that is very different from what I was used to in the West. In the United States we create breakthroughs in science or engineering at universities and in laboratories. We focus on mastering the tangible outer world. In India, however, there are countless rishis, yogis, and spiritual masters trying to create breakthroughs by mastering the inner world through consciousness, awakened intuition (the *third eye*), and exploration of metaphysical experiences. They use the tools of meditation, yoga, ancient healing methods, and *prana*, or life force. There are so many different faiths: different sects of Hinduism, Hare Krishna, Jainism, Sikhism, Islam, Buddhism, Christianity, Judaism, and too many more to name, with gurus and gods Westerners like me have never heard of. I met followers of all kinds of methods and teachers, including Osho, Sai Baba, Yogananda, Gurumayi, and Swaminarayan, all devoted to exploring the intangible supernatural existence beyond our minds. Passing a street vendor, I spontaneously bought a book I had never heard of that I later learned is well known, *Autobiography of a Yogi.* I was completely immersed in a new world that was stretching me beyond measure.

All the clean, clear lines we put around things in America blurred once I got to India. I was used to having a single God that looked a lot like an older and much wiser version of me, only with a beard and draped in white. In India, there were thousands of temples dedicated to hundreds of gods: one had the body of a human and the head of an elephant, one had blue skin, one looked like a monkey, one goddess had eight hands and rode on tigers, and that's just a few. In trying to make sense of it, a friend explained to me that although Hindus actually believe in only one God, they feel God cannot be contained by a single image. Having so many different versions of God expands humans into the realm of the spiritual which is beyond logic or reasoning and beyond the mind. The temples, mosques, and places of worship for various gods were everywhere, worked into busy street corners and shining in full majestic beauty on large plots of land with long queues of people waiting to enter. I was used to a sense of reverence and quiet in churches, but in Hindu temples, worship often entails bells, fire, and even shouting. There's a sense of anticipation, excitement, and fun. Like the festival Holi, where you throw multicolored chalk around until everyone is covered in a rainbow of colors from head to toe. It's exhilarating!

Alicia and I arrived in January 2010, when the weather was warm and mild. With so much to take in on our first trip to India, we were glad to escape into the peaceful green compound of Dr. Naram's clinic, a refuge from the traffic and congestion. The food at the café was amazing, combining flavors and textures I never imagined existed.

The staff were so kind, and I asked our waiter what it meant when I was speaking with Indians and they'd bob their head side to side. He affectionately called it the 'Indian head bob' and told me it could either mean "yes, I agree" or "no, I don't agree." I asked, "How can I tell the difference?" To which he replied, "I don't know." We all laughed. I decided it simply meant, "I acknowledge words are coming out of your mouth."

I came to India on an impulse and at considerable cost. In preparing for my trip, I rescheduled all the projects I was working on. In order for Alicia to join me, I used all the mileage points I had acquired to buy her ticket. I was anxiously excited to spend time with her.

I suppose it was also a huge risk for her, traveling to a foreign country with someone she barely knew. In India, though, she glowed more than usual, and I felt nervous around her. I wanted to impress her, but given my general social anxiety, all I could do was ask a lot of questions and answer very few. I consoled myself with the thought that even if it didn't work out between us, at least I helped make her dream trip come true.

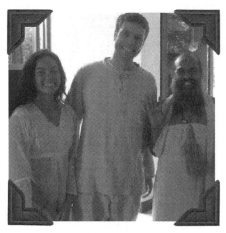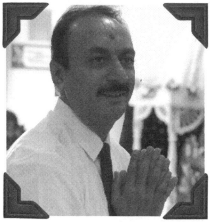

Left: Alicia, me, and Swami Omkar, whom we met at the clinic.
Right: Vinay Soni, Dr. Naram's kind-hearted administrative assistant.

When Dr. Naram arrived, there was a stir of excitement. Walking by his side was a tall man in a cream-colored shirt with a badge on the pocket I didn't recognize. He had a red dot on his forehead, surrounded by yellow marks. I discovered he was Vinay (pronounced *Veh-nay*), Dr. Naram's administrative assistant, whom I spoke with on the phone to arrange our visit. His countenance matched the humble and friendly tone of his voice.

Many of the people welcoming Dr. Naram had traveled from afar to be there and many did so in dire circumstances. Some were seeing him for the first time; others had known him for decades. As he walked through the crowd of people, his eyes met mine. He stopped and smiled as he pressed his hands together in front of his heart in a *namaste* pose. In response, I did the same, smiling because I remembered from our interview what that greeting meant. His friendly demeanor was a welcome relief from the nervousness I felt.

"Very happy you are here," he said. I introduced him to Alicia, who had a big smile on her face. Then he continued walking to his office to begin seeing patients.

When Your Life Is Like Hell

Whack! An eleven-year-old autistic girl named Gia (pronounced *Jee-uh*) just struck someone who was trying to calm her down. Sitting in front of Dr. Naram, her mother broke down into tears.

Alicia and I stood in Dr. Naram's office, which was packed with people. There were doctors from Germany, Italy, the United Kingdom, and Japan—all there to learn from him. There were staff members assisting and other patients waiting for their turn.

"I wish my daughter had never been born, Doctor. I know that sounds horrible, but it is true!" Gia's mother struggled to explain what her life was like raising a child like Gia. While she spoke, Dr. Naram quietly put his fingers on Gia's wrist until she yanked her hand away, knocking a box of mints off the desk. She jumped from her chair and bounced back and forth, from one side of the room to the other.

"My life is hell!" said Gia's mother. "We have no social life, no life. I spend every waking minute trying to make sure she doesn't hurt herself, us, or others. We cannot take her out in public, and I'm drained of every ounce of strength and attention just coping with her. She only wants to eat meat or junk food—she throws anything else we try to give her at us or on the floor. My relationship with my husband is tense. He is talking about leaving me. I snap at our other two children, who feel neglected, then get aggressive and make things even worse. I feel like a horrible wife and a failure as a mother."

Tears rolled down her cheeks as she hunched over in exhausted despair.

Dr. Naram patted her arm. "I'm not God," he said in a calm voice, "but I have helped thousands of children like this. The important thing is this question: 'What do you want?'"

There it is again, I thought. *That question.*

"I just want her to be a normal child, to have a normal life."

As she was speaking, Dr. Naram took notes on what he found in Gia's pulse. He quickly checked off boxes on a paper with names of various herbal formulas. He turned his bright, intense eyes back on the mother and said firmly, "What if we are able to make a transformation in Gia's life *and* yours right now?"

The mother stopped crying but also seemed to stop breathing. Before she could answer, Dr. Naram came from behind his desk and placed a chair in the middle of the room. "Gia," called Dr. Naram, patting the chair with his hand.

Everyone stared at him, except Gia.

She ignored him.

He walked to her and began to speak. She frantically bolted across the room, crashing into several people on the way. This happened several times. It seemed hopeless, and I wondered why he kept trying to do something that clearly wasn't going to work. This girl was too wild, and many other people were waiting to be seen.

Dr. Naram went to her again and tried to place his hands on her head in a particular way, to press certain points that he said activated a specific *marmaa*.

"Working with subtle energy points," he explained, "can help remove blocks and rebalance the body."

Only when he started to touch specific points on her head, Gia reached up and grabbed his face with her strong little hands. Her sharp nails scratched him, tearing the flesh on his left cheek. A few drops of bright red blood appeared on his dark skin. Dr. Naram jolted back in surprise.

"Gia!" her mom yelled in shock, vigorously trying to grab her daughter as she ran again across the room. Tension surged in my body as I watched Dr. Naram wipe the blood from his face with a tissue. Alicia looked terrified.

But the scratch startled Dr. Naram for only a brief moment. He began calling her name again.

"Gia."

When she didn't respond, her mother yelled her name again and tried to force her to sit on the chair.

"No!" Dr. Naram said abruptly to her mother. "Don't you understand? I'm trying to teach you something."

Tension permeated the room as the surprised mother let her child go. Gia watched her mother being scolded, then rushed to the other side of the room. She picked up the box of mints from the floor and started looking at it with great curiosity.

Dr. Naram joined her. "Very interesting, huh?"

She tapped it, so he tapped it.

Her mother tried to grab her hand to yank the box away. Again Dr. Naram said firmly, "No. I'm trying to teach you something. Don't you understand me?"

Gia looked at Dr. Naram, then went back to examining the box. Dr. Naram laughed and, smiling, said, "She is curious."

Then, turning to the little girl, he said, "I like you, Gia. I like how you're curious."

They explored the box together. He opened it, took a mint, and gave her one. After a short exchange, he was able to gently put his hands on her head and do the first marmaa. With the palm of his right hand on her forehead, the palm of his left hand on the back of her head, and his fingers curled and pressing lightly on the top of her head, he gave six squeezes. He took her right hand and pressed the tip of her index finger six times. Gia looked up at him inquisitively. She did not resist.

I was surprised. *Was this the big thing that was supposed to bring about a change? How on earth could squeezing the girl's head and pressing points on her hand help?*

When Dr. Naram went to press the third marmaa, a spot between the nose and the upper lip, Gia pushed his hand away and ran into the corner of the room. He patiently went to her and started from the beginning, with the first marmaa, then the second, soothing her with his voice. When he tried to do the third marmaa this time, she reluctantly let him.

"You are a very good girl, Gia" he said.

As she watched, he walked over to the empty chair, tapped it with his hand six times, and called her name. She yanked her gaze away from him and focused on the box in her hands. He went over again and repeated the three marmaas in sequence several times, speaking softly and kindly all the while.

"Now, Gia, when you come with me over to this chair, everyone in this room is going to acknowledge you and give you a big round of applause."

He gently took her hand and said firmly, "Now, come with me, Gia!"

She followed him to the chair and sat right on it.

We all started clapping. For the first time, Gia looked around at the people in the room through her thick glasses and gave us a huge smile. Dr. Naram was beaming, too.

He tapped her with his right hand over her heart and said, "Very good, Gia!"

Dr. Naram then patted another chair, but she didn't move toward it. Instead, she headed straight back to the box again.

He patiently repeated the marmaa points and said, "Now, come here, Gia." This time she went to the new chair and sat down. Everyone clapped, and Gia smiled an even bigger smile.

Again, Dr. Naram patted her over her heart six times, speaking words of encouragement. "Very good, Gia! Now come and meet Dr. Giovanni, and then come back and sit on your chair."

As Dr. Naram spoke, he demonstrated to Gia what he meant by going over to Dr. Giovanni and shaking his hand, then returned to the chair. She looked confused. Again, Dr. Naram did the three marmaas on her in sequence. He repeated the demonstration several times, then did the marmaa sequence once more.

This time, he held her hand and she followed him to Dr. Giovanni, shook his hand, then triumphantly sat on her chair amid applause. He proceeded to have her do the same and shake the hand of one of the clinic's patients, a man by the name of Paul Suri who had come from New Jersey. Paul was very encouraging to Gia. Then, Dr. Naram surprised me.

"Now, come meet Dr. Clint." Dr. Naram demonstrated coming over to me and shaking my hand.

It was enough to show her once. Gia came straight over, shook my hand, and something deep inside me melted. She smiled so big at me I couldn't help but smile back. I looked at Alicia, who was beaming with joy. Everyone was clapping and smiling, except Gia's mother. She was in tears. "I . . . I don't understand."

Dr. Naram said, "It is important to remember that Gia doesn't actually care for *your* understanding, and she doesn't care for your tears, either. She cares for *her* understanding! Marmaa is an ancient technology of transformation. Through these marmaas, you can communicate messages that go directly to the subconscious in a way that *she can feel understood.* When you combine this with a certain diet, herbal remedies, and home remedies—amazing things can happen. I have seen it work now on thousands of children, with great results, over thirty years. She will listen to you, obey you, and become happy and healthy."

Dr. Naram asked Dr. Giovanni to take Gia and her mother into a separate room to teach her the marmaa points, to explain the diet, and to answer any questions about the herbal formulas he prescribed for her.

As Dr. Giovanni opened the door, Dr. Naram spotted a familiar family waiting in the hall. He stopped everything to welcome them into the room and gave the young father a big hug. "Whenever I see this man, I feel it is better than winning a Nobel Prize!" he exclaimed.

Looking at Gia's mother, Dr. Naram said, "When I first met this man about fifteen years ago, he was far worse off than your daughter. His mother had lost all hope." He motioned to the elderly mother, who also entered the room, and then put his hand on the young man's shoulder.

"He couldn't dress himself or speak more than a few mumbled words. And drooled on himself all the time. All his mother wanted was for him to be a normal boy. And after years of work, you see this boy grew into a man!"

The elderly mother spoke up: "He still is not 100 percent."

Dr. Naram said, "Yes, but look now. After all these years of following the deeper healing secrets, his brain grew! And believe it or not, this boy who once couldn't say his own name is now married and has a job. He is supporting a home with his wife and a brilliant daughter." Dr. Naram pointed at his wife and daughter standing next to him, adding, "His daughter is now doing schoolwork so well that she is in the top of her class!"

"Look," Dr. Naram said to the elderly mother, "your son is happily married with a wife *and* has a beautiful daughter. Now look at Dr. Giovanni; it is difficult for us to even get him married." Everyone laughed, including Dr. Giovanni.

Dr. Naram looked at Gia's mother and said, "Please talk with this family. Be inspired by what is possible if you really choose to follow the ancient secrets of deeper healing. It takes time, patience, commitment, and effort, but amazing things are possible."

He then turned to me. "Dr. Clint, you must also talk with them to hear their full story."

I followed the two families and Dr. Giovanni into another room. I felt compelled to record the incredible story of this young father and his beautiful family.

Later, researching online, I was shocked to read that, according to the US Center for Disease Control and Prevention (CDC), there has been a 600 percent increase in autism rates in the last twenty years! I discovered that one out of seventy boys is diagnosed with autism in the United States alone. That number does not include the millions of other children who are increasingly diagnosed with attention deficit disorder (ADD/ADHD) and other developmental or social disorders. Having seen Gia for only a few minutes, I pondered what life was like for each of those families. Looking into the solutions available to them, I couldn't find any mention of the ancient healing methods Dr. Naram was using. I learned only that while Western medicine has no cure for autism, most of these children are given some form of prescription drugs, many of which have troubling side effects. Reviewing the video and notes I'd captured, I wondered how many people could benefit from the ancient healing method Dr. Naram was using.*

Bonus Material: For more context about how Dr. Naram would help someone with ADD/ADHD or autism, please refer to the videos in the free MyAncientSecrets.com membership site. As always, please remember the medical disclaimer.

A Global Attraction

Alicia and I spent as much time as we could at the clinic. Hundreds of people came each day, and Dr. Naram often stayed well past midnight. Sitting in the cafeteria or walking in the halls, I began asking patients and foreign doctors about their experiences. I wanted to hear from the doctors why they'd come. I wondered why patients traveled so far to spend only five to ten minutes with Dr. Naram. In a single week, I counted patients from eighty-five countries!

Midway through the week, I documented more and more of my conversations by video, recording interviews with patients and taking pictures of their medical reports when they would let me. The more I heard and saw, the more surprised I was that no one had captured these stories already. I felt the recordings would make a nice thank-you gift to Dr. Naram for letting us join him. It also gave me something to do other than hope Alicia was starting to like me.

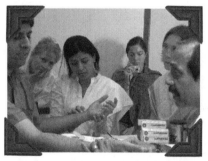

Alicia taking a picture of the activity happening in Dr. Naram's office.

The range of ailments people claimed Dr. Naram helped them with was astounding—everything from joint pain to infertility, skin disease, hormonal imbalances, heart disease, hydrocephalus, mental conditions, and even cancer. Hearing this, one question kept nagging me. *Doctors in the United States usually focus on one area of speciality (like a heart specialist or a urologist); how was it possible for Dr. Naram to achieve such great results in so many areas?* I still wondered, *Was it all just placebo effect?*

I discovered that even though the conditions varied greatly, the solution for each usually included changing habits, starting with diet, and it took time before patients saw results. Many confessed that they tried other methods in search of a quick fix before coming to Dr. Naram. All too often, these quick-fix solutions came with an array of long-term side effects. They told me the ancient healing methods of Dr. Naram took more time but brought real, long-term, and deeper healing results with no negative side effects.

On the third day, a young couple brought their ten-year-old daughter, who had never spoken in her life. Dr. Naram worked with her for about ten minutes, pressing certain points on her body while asking her to respond. With the entire room watching with tense anticipation, this little girl spurted out "Mommy!" The room erupted in applause as the obvious delight showed on this little girl's face and in her eyes. She said "Mommy" again, and when I looked over at her mother, I saw she was in tears.

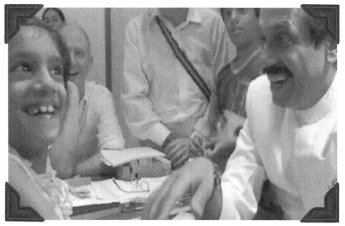

*Screenshot from video—the moment immediately after
this little girl said "Mommy" for the first time.*

Some people told me they had known Dr. Naram for more than thirty-five years and felt like they were part of his family. Others knew him more recently, spending only five minutes with him, but still had profound results during the subsequent months of taking his healing herbs, home remedies, and/or changing their diet. I was amazed that teachers from so many different spiritual traditions sent their students and devotees to Dr. Naram for help. Some came for cures for physical illness and others to detoxify their bodies, preparing their minds so they could deepen their meditation practice and spiritual experience.

I was intrigued but had no idea what to make of it all. Despite the remarkable things I saw, I became increasingly irritable. It was becoming painfully clear that things between Alicia and me were not going to progress beyond friendship. I was getting subtle cues that although she was grateful to be having this experience, she was not interested in me. I felt a combination of frustration, sadness, and resignation.

Unexpected Remedy

On our last day at the clinic, Dr. Naram asked to speak with me after he finished seeing patients. Excited as I was to talk with him, by the time our meeting came, at 1:30 a.m., a throbbing headache made it tough for me to focus.

"Can I ask you a question?" I said when we finally sat down. "How can I get rid of this headache? I've been eating healthy, exercising, and even had a therapeutic massage today. I don't even know where it came from."

His dark, curious eyes focused in on me. "Where does it hurt?"

Focusing in on the source point of the pain, I pointed to the base of my head and neck.

"Ahh. That is a *vata* headache." I never knew there were different kinds of headaches, which you could identify by where your head was hurting.

"For that kind of headache, your medicine is . . . onion rings."

"What? Onion rings?" *Did I hear him correctly?*

Dr. Naram smiled. "The original master of my Siddha-Veda lineage, Jivaka, taught how everything can be either a poison or a medicine, depending on how you use it. For example, water is a medicine for ninety-two conditions and a poison for twenty-six. Even the things you do, like your work, can be a medicine or a poison, depending on whether it is aligned with your life's purpose or not."

He explained patiently, yet with an intensity and enthusiasm I wouldn't have expected from someone who had seen over three hundred patients that day.

"There are three main kinds of headaches and lots of different subtypes. Onion rings won't work for *every* type of headache. Also, if you eat them all the time, they will create toxins in your body. So, for long-term, deeper healing I can tell you what else to do. But for your headache right now, eating onion rings is a temporary medicine. Just test it out for yourself."

Dr. Naram asked the chef who was still there to make some fresh onion *pakoda* (pronounced *pah-koh-dah*; an Indian dish similar to onion rings). My head was throbbing.

"Everything can be either a poison or a medicine, depending on how you use it."

–Jivaka (Ancient physician of Buddha)

As I put the deliciously cooked onions in my mouth, I was curious what would happen. To my shock and awe, the pain, which had been growing in intensity all day, quickly began to drain from my body and completely disappeared within five minutes.

"That's amazing!" I told Dr. Naram. With my headache gone and my heart opening I asked him, "How did that work?"

"You know Clint, you remind me a lot of myself when I was younger."

"Really? How so?" I was intrigued to know how we might be the same.

"I was also messed up and confused," he said with a laugh.

My face was blank. Dr. Naram smiled and put his hand on my arm. He described how his master helped him gain tremendous clarity in his life, teaching him lost ancient secrets for transformation and deep healing.

"Onions are one of so many powerful medicines from nature. There are many secrets like this that I can teach you. They may shock you at first, but they can change your life forever. What is more, once you know them, you become a powerful influence on this planet to help others!"

I considered my visit to India to be a one-time event, and soon I'd be going back to my work in technology research at the university. I wondered why he was telling me this. I thought, *Shouldn't Alicia be here for this conversation instead of me?* When I walked outside the door I saw her learning more about how to read pulses from Dr. Giovanni, so I felt satisfied she was also getting whatever she needed. It was late, but Dr. Naram asked to talk with me once more before I left India, inviting Alicia and me to his home for a meal.

When I got to my bedroom, I realized that along with the

headache, also the frustration from the day had melted away. That night I was left with a sense of awe. As I reflected on everything, my thoughts drifted to Alicia and then back to Dr. Naram. He had a way of helping me forget my inadequacies and self-perceived limitations. He opened me up to a world of new possibilities. And he taught me such a cool remedy for the kind of headache that I had!

My Journal Notes

Ancient Healing Secrets for a Vata Headache*

1) Determine the type of headache: According to Dr. Naram, if pain is in the front of the head, sinus areas, it is likely a Kapha headache. If the pain is sharp on the top, or on one side, it is likely a Pitta headache. If the pain is on the back, or base of neck, it is likely a Vata headache.

2) If it is a Vata headache, you can give these ancient remedies:
    a) Home Remedy—Eat a few onion rings* or onion pakoda (an Indian dish of fried onions)
    b) Marmaa Shakti—Four fingers down from the earlobes on each side of the neck, press 6 times.

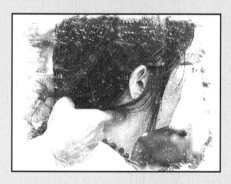

*Important: Dr. Naram only recommended the above remedy for a specific type of headache, and did not recommend people take onion rings every day to 'prevent headaches', either, because it would be toxic for your body.

Bonus Material: To see how Dr. Naram would help several common types of headache, please visit the free MyAncientSecrets.com membership site.

The next day, I decided to research Dr. Naram's lineage. There wasn't much information available in English on Master Jivaka, but I did find one well-documented story. It told how Buddha (Siddhartha Gautama) had summoned all the physicians and healers and given them a test. He asked them to go into the forest and come back with a bag full of everything they found that was not useful for healing. Some came back proud of their huge bags, saying they had no use for any of these particular plants. Others came back with smaller bags. Only one came back with nothing. When questioned by Buddha, Jivaka responded that he was not able to find a single thing that was not useful for a health condition. That is when Buddha requested that Jivaka be his physician.

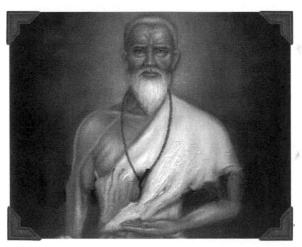

Illustration of Master Jivaka. Retrieved from Google Images.

Whenever Buddha would travel, Jivaka traveled with him, helping to care for the entourage and all those who came in search of enlightenment. On his many journeys, Jivaka discovered new plants and new uses for them. He recorded his findings in manuscripts that have been preserved for centuries.

Reading this story made me smile. It seemed Dr. Naram took the lesson to heart, that everything was useful in healing—even onion rings.

As I lay in bed, I wondered if Dr. Naram knew any ancient healing secrets that could help me overcome rejection and heartache.

Your Journal Notes

To deepen and magnify the benefits you will experience from reading this book, take a few minutes now and answer the following questions for yourself:

What thoughts, conversations, foods, and/or activities feel like poison in your life? (Decreasing your vital energy)

_____

_____

_____

_____

What thoughts, conversations, foods, and/or activities feel like medicine in your life? (Increasing your vital energy)

_____

_____

_____

_____

What other insights, questions, or realizations came to you as you read this chapter?

_____

_____

_____

_____

CHAPTER 4

What Matters Most?

You could go up to almost anyone and instead of asking
"How are you?" you could ask "Where does it hurt?"

–Henry B. Eyring

Remember that call from my father I mentioned in the introduction to this book? The next morning was when that happened.

I couldn't miss the subdued but palpable distress in his voice. "Son, can you come home? I need to talk to you."

When I asked my dad what was happening, he wouldn't say. He only emphasized that he needed to speak with me in person.

"How soon can you make it to Utah?" he asked.

As it happened, Alicia and I would be flying out the next night. She was returning to California and I was going to New York, then on to Utah, where my parents lived. For the rest of the day, thoughts of my father filled my mind.

So you can understand us better, I want to share a bit about my dad and our family. My parents raised eight kids—a houseful. I was their sixth child, but I enjoyed telling people I was their favorite. At school a friend once asked me, "Why are there so many kids in your family—didn't your parents have a TV?"

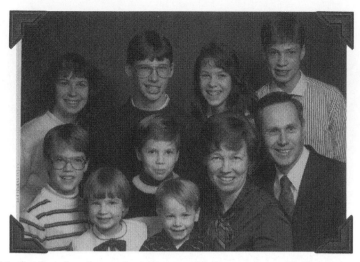

My family when I was about 6 years old; I'm center, my dad and mom on the right front, and my sister Denise is the top left corner.

Most of the time, I loved having so many brothers and sisters. Sure we fought about silly things, but we also laughed a lot and knew how to play and create. I remember one of my older brothers brought home a video camera one day and we got hooked on making funny videos. Losing my oldest sister, Denise, to suicide brought the rest of us closer together. One thing we didn't do well was talk about our feelings, but we knew how much we cared for one another without ever saying it.

My parents were faithfully married for more than forty years, through the thick and thin of life. When my dad proposed to my mom, he said, "Knowing what you know about me, will you still be the mother of my children?" I always thought that was a funny way to propose to her.

Though they never had much money, they made ends meet. I loved getting a box full of hand-me-down clothes from a neighbor or family from church. I still remember when I found out that most people went to the store and paid a lot of money for clothes, and how strange that seemed to me. My parents taught us the value of frugality, hard work, prayer, honesty, and commitment.

Mom and Dad were very different. My mom liked to get things

done, with a talent for putting people into action. I was amazed by how efficient she was and by how much she accomplished each day. I suppose that in order to raise eight kids, you'd have to develop that skill. My dad, on the other hand, was more concerned about how everyone was feeling than what they were doing.

My dad's passion was helping parents and teachers understand what he called "the missing piece in education." The missing piece, he felt, was we teach kids in school *what* to think, but not *how* to think. He had a motto that "a single idea can change a child's life." Inspired by Benjamin Franklin, he loved integrating ethics with education, teaching kids to develop character while simultaneously helping them learn any subject better. His dream was to synthesize the thirty plus years of his life's work into a book he would call *The Missing Piece in Education*, as his legacy to his grandchildren. For that, Dad always had a stack of papers on his desk, compiling engaging questions, activities and stories that helped guide children how to think, and how to make good choices. In my most honest moments, I wished I was more adept at that.

Dad had a funny, self-effacing sense of humor. When I was little and learning how to tie my shoe laces, I asked him, "Dad, can you put my shoes on?" He replied with a smile, "Yeah, I can try, but I'm not sure they'll fit me." Then he'd gently teach me how to tie my own shoes. When one of us walked up behind him and gave him a shoulder massage, he'd say, "I'll give you exactly two hours to cut that out."

We laughed so much! For example, one time my dad was saying the family prayer at night and fell asleep halfway through. We sat there waiting, confused. The best part was that when he told the story, he couldn't help but burst out laughing at himself. He laughed so hard he'd cry at how funny the whole thing was, and we cracked up with him. He taught me that laughter is one of the most powerful medicines for any person or family. As much as he loved laughing, he'd never laugh at the expense of others and stopped us if we did. He taught me by example that if we could laugh at ourselves and our own mistakes, it was somehow easier to move past them.

> "A single idea can change a child's life."
> –George L. Rogers

> *"Laughter is one of the most powerful medicines for any person or family."*
>
> –George L. Rogers

People loved being around him. As a teenager, my friends told me how much they felt he cared about them. When I was about sixteen years old, a friend surprised me by saying, "Your dad is so easy to be with. I look in his eyes and I just feel loved."

He was kind but strong. He would not compromise when it came to a principle he believed in. One year when I was about twelve, he discovered I was going to illegally copy music and videos to give to my mom and grandma as Christmas gifts; it made perfect sense to me as a way to save money! I could tell how strongly he disapproved when he found out. He told me people who created the music and videos should get paid. He said, "Never do anything you would be ashamed of if it became public." Then, understanding I didn't have much money, he took me to the store and added to the money I had, so I could afford the video and music I had wanted to copy. He corrected me, yet in a way that made me feel good about myself.

Understanding and appreciating my mom was more difficult and complicated until later in life. Because I was a sensitive kid, I noticed there were frequently things under the surface that troubled her. I didn't know what they were, or whether some of them were my fault, because she never spoke about them, at least not to me. Instead, she would thrust herself into nonstop work and "to-do" lists as a way to maintain a sense of control and accomplishment, somehow keeping a family of eight kids functioning.

> *"Never do anything you would be ashamed of if it became public."*
>
> –George L. Rogers

In addition to being sensitive, I was also shy and easily took things personally. When I was nine years old, I was so angry at my mom when I overheard her on the phone with one of her friends, laughing while sharing an embarrassing story about me. For something that other kids might have ignored or laughed along with, I felt hurt and violated. *She was supposed to love me, not laugh about me to others.* I blamed the pain I felt on her and wanted her to hurt also. I'm ashamed to admit that, but it's true. Initially I wanted to run away, but I decided to stay home and give her the silent treatment. It lasted about a day and a half, until she came into my room the next evening.

"Clint, what's happening?" she asked. "I can't help you if I don't know what's wrong."

I tried my best not to talk, and eventually broke into tears. She reached out and tenderly rubbed my back, showing so much compassion that I couldn't hold her as a monster in my mind anymore. I confessed why I was hurting. She immediately apologized and hugged me tightly.

Don't get me wrong. I had frustrations with my dad, too. I got upset when he confronted me about doing something wrong, like the time I hit my sister. She was in tears. Firmly pulling me away, he sat me on the stairs and asked, "Why did you hit your sister?"

I felt totally justified sharing my reason, "Because she made me mad."

He paused and said something that changed my life. "Son, no one can *make* you mad, or *make* you feel anything. Your reaction always comes from inside you. People can control your emotions only if you allow them to."

Even though he still punished me for hitting my sister, the truth of his wisdom hit me deeper. It was an *aha* moment that melted away the anger I felt. He was right: no one could make me mad. I was responsible for my own emotions. It was an amazing discovery.

> *"No one can make you mad. Your reaction always comes from inside you."*
>
> –George L. Rogers

Priceless Kindness

While I was in India, my dad's call stirred a lot of memories like these. Later that day, I saw Vinay, Dr. Naram's administrative assistant.

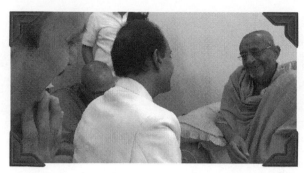

Dr. Naram just after taking the pulse of Hariprasad Swamijii,
a spiritual master for millions who promotes the concept of Atmiyata.
Vinay looking at both of them with love and devotion.

Seeing the distant look on my face, he asked, "Are you okay?"

"Not really," I said. "I'm worried about my dad."

I told him about the call, and then shared some stories about my father. Vinay said, "I'm amazed. Your father is following a principle I learned from my spiritual master, Hariprasad Swamijii, called *Atmiyata*" (pronounced *Aht-me-yah-tah*).

"What's that?"

"Essentially, the concept of Atmiyata is that you treat people with love and respect, no matter how they treat you. I'm pleased to learn that people like your dad follow such a principle. That's different than what we see on the TV and in movies about American culture."

I agreed that my dad had a strong, clear conscience, and I admired him for it. I always felt like I had a lot to live up to. At the same time, I quietly felt like I was failing to live up to his example.

What I didn't tell Vinay was that I often felt the weight of poor choices I made that I was ashamed of. I never told my parents about several of them and hoped they'd never find out. I didn't want to disappoint them.

In the hopes of making my parents and family proud of me instead, I accomplished many things. I graduated at the top of my high school class, spoke at our graduation commencement ceremony, and was accepted on scholarship to a great university. I did a lot of service work in Africa and other parts of the world, postponed part of university to do missionary work for two years, and went on to be the first in my family to get a PhD with award-winning dissertation research. I received several awards and acknowledgements as a young researcher. I was even chosen as one of twelve young scholars from around the world to be flown to Brussels for

> *"Atmiyata is when, no matter how someone treats you, you can respond with love and respect."*
>
> –Hariprasad Swamijii

a "meeting of young masterminds" discussing potential solutions to world problems. At that time, I was based in Finland, coordinating a European Union–funded project. I taught pioneering courses on how to use technology and new media for interfaith/intercultural communication, international development, and peace-building efforts. Despite all that, the mistakes I made, in my mind, outweighed anything good I'd done.

When my dad called that morning and said he needed to see me, for a moment I wondered if he had discovered something I'd done wrong.

In addition to supporting me, I knew my parents worried about me, as parents do. And I knew they prayed for me a lot. I traveled to and lived in different countries but was nowhere close to getting married. I was exploring my own relationship with spirituality and science, spending a lot of time far away from home and from everything they were familiar with. I once confided in my dad that I felt sad and lonely, so he always made sure to ask me how I was and if things were getting better. I think he took extra care because of what had happened with my sister. I endeavored to stay in close touch with them, but that call from my dad and his request to meet came out of the blue.

It was unusual for him to set up an appointment with me. I was his son and he could call me anytime. All day I was confused, then even more concerned when my mom called later that evening.

"Please don't forget the meeting with your father," my mom said with a tone in her voice I wasn't used to. "I don't know what it's about, but I feel it's important."

The mystery would have to wait. I had another day in Mumbai and then a stop in New York before I'd find out what my dad needed.

And before I left India, Dr. Naram requested to meet with me once more to share something he said would change my life.

Your Journal Notes

To deepen and magnify the benefits you will experience from reading this book, take a few minutes now and answer the following questions for yourself:

What hidden struggles are those you love facing right now? What might you be able to do to help them?

_____

_____

_____

What wisdom have you learned from your parents or others, which has helped you?

_____

_____

_____

Where is an area of your life where you can practice the healing art of Atmiyata?

_____

_____

_____

What other insights, questions, or realizations came to you as you read this chapter?

_____

_____

_____

CHAPTER 5

A Great Secret for Succeeding at Anything

When we no longer know what to do, we have come to our real work and when we no longer know which way to go, we have begun our real journey.

–Wendell Berry

The next night, before Alicia and I would take a red-eye flight to the United States, Dr. Naram hosted us for a farewell meal. Although the food was delicious, I ate quickly, hoping to have more time to talk with him. Finally, he said, "Could you meet me alone in my study? I want to show you something very special."

Once I closed the door of the study behind me, Dr. Naram brought out several bundles wrapped in orange cloth. As he untied the string around them, I saw they contained old, worn pages covered with handwritten characters I did not recognize. In a hushed tone, Dr. Naram said, "These are some pages from the ancient texts given to me by my master." He carefully handled each page, sharing how precious the manuscripts were to him and how they guided him to the ancient principles, formulas, and methods he used to help people.

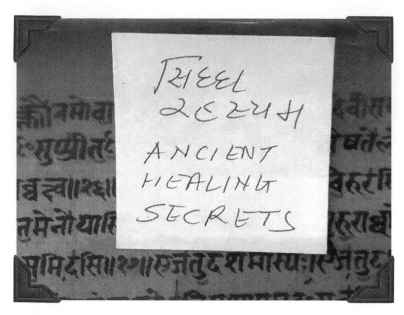

Ancient manuscripts containing ancient healing secrets.

A scrap of yellow paper at the beginning of each text, written in English, provided a short description of the contents. They were written in several languages: Sanskrit, Tibetan, Nerali, Nepali, and Ardhamagadhi or Magadhi Prakrit. There were home remedies and herbal formulas for diabetes, different kinds of cancer, and hair and skin problems and ancient mantras and marmaas for manifesting happiness, peace, and abundance. There were even secret youth formulas used by a lady called Amrapali who, Dr. Naram explained, was over sixty years old but looked thirty years younger. She was so attractive that a thirty-five-year-old king fell in love with her despite already having a beautiful young wife. I had a strong desire to touch these ancient writings, but I didn't want to risk damaging the fragile paper.

"My whole life has been about following the instructions of my master," Dr. Naram said, "so that I could decode the principles from these ancient pages and bring them into physical reality in the modern world in a way that changes and even saves people's lives."

There was a long pause as I let those words sink in. Breaking the silence, I asked him a question that was burning inside me for a while: "Where did this all start for you?"

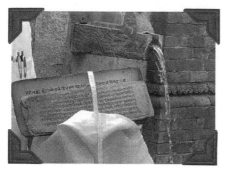 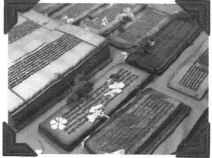

Left: Dr. Naram holding one of the ancient texts containing his lineage's secrets for deeper and deeper healing. Right: More manuscripts on a table.

As he tenderly rewrapped the ancient pages in the orange cloth, Dr. Naram told me his story.

"Thirty years ago, I had graduated from university as a doctor."

"What? Before becoming a healer, you were trained as a doctor?"

"Yes, I graduated with a bachelor's degree in 1978 from Bombay University, and advanced Ayurvedic medical degrees in 1982 and 1984. Only thing is, I was still a doctor from nowhere. I had a big dream of wanting to change the world. I wanted to help people attain vibrant health, peace of mind, and unlimited energy, but I had no energy, health, or peace myself. What is more, despite all my education, I was still working with only a 'maybe theory.' Do you know what a 'maybe theory' is?"

I shrugged and shook my head.

"Suppose a patient came and said he had a stomach ache. I'd say, 'Maybe gas, maybe acidity, or maybe some tumor,' or 'Maybe some problem with his wife.' I'd give a broad spectrum of remedies based on 'maybe' guesses, and he'd go away. He would come back with the same problem a month later and I'd say, 'Maybe it is psychosomatic.' I'd spend hours consulting with my patients without getting results. I was frustrated, depressed, nervous, and anxious. I felt like a failure. I ate bad food to calm my anxiety and gained lots of weight. I was over 220 pounds and beginning to question whether the remedies I was using were effective. Or maybe the problem was that I did not understand people. Maybe I didn't understand their real challenges, concerns, fears, and anxieties. Maybe this was not a job for me."

As Dr. Naram spoke about not being happy, I reflected on my own sadness. It was not always there, but it came frequently enough to make me question many things in my life. Sometimes it appeared as depression; sometimes as impatience, or irritation with myself and others.

"I was not making any money and had no job satisfaction—no inside joy," Dr. Naram continued, "Then, one day, a miracle changed my life forever. I was treating a patient named Shanker (pronounced *Shawn-ker*). He came every week, and we sat together for two hours discussing his problem and trying new solutions and remedies, but nothing worked. Suddenly, after two years of meeting, Shanker stopped coming, and I thought, maybe I finally cured someone. Several months later, I saw him walking down the road looking happy. I wondered, *Did I help him?* His answer shook me to the core.

"Shanker told me, 'No, Dr. Naram, you did not help me. No matter how much time you took, you never understood me. You just confused me more and more.' I replied, 'I know my problem is that I don't understand people! So how did you get better?'"

Shanker explained that he'd gone to a great master who was 115 years old. The man touched his pulse and, in only two minutes, told him exactly what was happening in his body, mind, and emotions and advised him what to do to heal. Dr. Naram didn't believe this was possible, but there was no denying that Shanker looked much better. His medical reports showed dramatic improvements in diabetes, arthritis, blood pressure, osteoporosis, and kidney function. Dr. Naram asked, "How can I meet this master and see for myself?"

"Shanker gave me the location," Dr. Naram continued, "But before going, I made a list of all my problems: depression, anxiety, nervousness, diabetes, hair loss, and obesity. Then I traveled to this great master and waited a long time in line before it was my turn. All the while, I pondered how this 115-year-old man was still seeing ninety clients a day. When it was finally my turn, the healer put his fingers on the pulse of my wrist and said: 'High blood sugar. Also, you want to grow hair, lose weight, and you want to change your

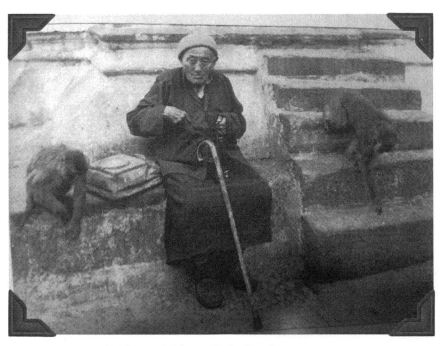

Dr. Naram's Master, Baba Ramdas, at age 115.

job. In addition you are depressed, nervous, and confused about the future.'"

Dr. Naram paused for a moment. "He understood me, and I can't tell you how good it felt to be deeply understood like that. Later my master told me, 'In the last six thousand years of human history, the greatest need people have is not love, but understanding.'"

As Dr. Naram shared his story, I wondered: *In addition to helping people with things like high blood pressure, diabetes, arthritis, and so on, did that master also have ancient secrets that could turn sadness into happiness?*

Dr. Naram continued, "Baba Ramdas understood me, and that single meeting changed my life. I was given a prescription for some herbs and some diet changes and was asked to come again in six months. The master told me that he had no quick fix for me. If that is what I wanted, I should go somewhere else. What he was offering was deeper healing that required persistence and patience. I did exactly as he told me. It took time but my patience

"In the last six thousand years of human history, the greatest need people have is not love, but understanding."

–Baba Ramdas
(Dr. Naram's Master)

and commitment paid off. The prescription worked like magic. I lost weight, from 220 pounds to now 127 pounds. My blood sugar level dropped significantly, from 475 when fasting to now 96 to 105 when fasting. And my hair grew back. When I started I had lots of time but no hair. Now I have lots of hair but no time."

We both smiled. As I listened to his story, I said, "Wow ... what a gift."

"Yes, but do you know what the greatest gift he gave me was?"

"What?"

"He taught me, in a way I will never forget, the greatest secret to understanding ourselves and others. And he also taught me the secret to succeeding at anything."

Understanding Ourselves to Understand Others

Dr. Naram explained how meeting this master instilled in him a desire to learn everything about ancient healing secrets. He thought that learning them was a way to prove to his father and friends that he was not a miserable failure. He could show them he was doing something worthwhile and not wasting his life.

"So I went to this great master and said, 'I would like to learn this secret art and science of pulse healing.'

"Baba Ramdas said, 'Very good. Come tomorrow.'

"So I went tomorrow, and said again to him, 'I would like to learn this secret art and science of pulse healing.' Then he said, 'Come tomorrow.' He kept saying he would teach me 'tomorrow,' so I did come tomorrow ... for a hundred days!"

Dr. Naram recounted that it was thoroughly confusing and that, on the hundredth day, he decided he had enough. So he made a commitment: *If he doesn't teach me today, I will stand in front of him like a rock. I will die, but I will not move.*

He stood in front of Baba Ramdas and told him, "I've come to learn and won't leave until you agree to teach me."

Baba Ramdas said, "Who decides?"

"I decide," Dr. Naram said.

"That is your problem," Baba Ramdas replied.

Dr. Naram stood in front of the 115-year-old master like a rock for hours. "It was amazing how, while he was seeing the patients, he was also watching me. As I stood there, I saw him touch their pulse and then read them like a book, one after another. Finally, after four hours I obviously needed badly to go to the bathroom. He saw me wiggling my body and squeezing my legs to try to hold it, and said, 'Dr. Naram, I think you would like to go to the bathroom.' I said, 'Yes.' He said, 'Then go to the bathroom.' I said, 'But I would like to learn from you.' He said, 'Then come tomorrow.'"

The way Dr. Naram told the story, with his gestures and facial expressions, made me laugh.

He looked at me and said, "You may laugh, but I started to cry. And in that moment, something must have happened to this master. He said, 'OK, stop crying.' I said, 'What do I do?' He said, 'Come, today your training starts.' With some hope and surprise, I said, 'What should I do first?' He answered, 'Go to the bathroom.' So I went to the bathroom right away. I came back and said, 'OK, what should I do to start my training?' This great master asked me, 'How many people have used the bathroom today so far?' I guessed, 'Maybe thirty to forty?' He said, 'Very good. Go clean the bathroom.'"

This confused Dr. Naram. After all, he was a doctor, and this was below him. Dr. Naram told Baba Ramdas, "Sir, I think you must have misunderstood. I came to learn pulse healing, not bathroom cleaning."

Baba Ramdas quickly replied, "Oh, you want to learn pulse healing. No problem, come tomorrow."

And so the young Dr. Naram promptly went to clean the bathroom.

"Only later I understood that Baba Ramdas first needed to break my ego and help me face my fears. This was the greatest gift he could have ever given me. This is one secret. Our two greatest obstacles in life (to seeing ourselves or others clearly) are ego and fear. If we have a big ego or fears, we cannot see what is happening in a patient's body, mind, and emotions. Ego and fears prevent us from seeing ourselves clearly, so how can we see what is happening in those who come to us? We cannot feel what they are feeling or understand what they are experiencing. We can't truly understand ourselves or anyone else until we are able to face our ego and fears. Until then, our vision is clouded and blurry. Baba Ramdas told me, 'Healer, first heal thyself,' and my healing started with cleaning toilets."

Hearing his story, I began to question:

How does my own ego affect me?
How do my fears impact my life?
How do both blind me to not see myself or others clearly?
How do they influence the way I am—in relationships, with my family,
    at work, or in my spiritual life?

I recalled an experience I had a few months before the trip to India. I was running a European Union project at my university in Finland and was suitably proud of it. I was the only American and the youngest researcher reporting at meetings in Brussels. However, not everyone felt good about my role. A graduate student from the Netherlands wrote me a bitter email to tell me how much he disliked the way I was handling my duties.

I felt misunderstood and angry. *Everyone else was complimenting me, so what was wrong with this guy?* Instead of listening and asking more questions to understand his point of view, I attacked him by pointing out the ways in which his argument was shortsighted, trying to invalidate his opinion. I told him that some people on the project were dissatisfied with the contributions he was being paid for.

Not only did I miss an opportunity to learn something about myself and improve the project, I failed to see him clearly. Only later did I discover he was depressed and experiencing a personal life low. Instead of being part of the solution in his life, I magnified the problem.

"Our two greatest obstacles in life (to seeing ourselves or others clearly) are ego and fear."

–Dr. Naram

Listening to Dr. Naram, I contemplated how many times in my life I failed to see things clearly because of my fears and ego. Looking back, I realized just how confused and insecure I often felt, wanting people to like me, wanting to appear more successful than I was. I would even lie about stupid things to try and influence someone's perception of me, or hide a mistake I made. All these things were by-products of the deeper issues: fear and ego.

I asked myself:

How would my life be different if I wasn't influenced by my fear and ego?
How would I change for the better?

"So many people from around the world admire you," I said to Dr. Naram. "How do you keep your ego from clouding your judgment in the midst of so much praise? And with situations in which your reputation is at stake, how do you keep from being afraid?"

"I'd be lying if I said fear and ego didn't still come and go," Dr. Naram replied. "When Gia, the girl with severe autism, scratched me and I started to bleed while everyone was watching, I was nervous for a moment. I wasn't certain that my ancient secrets would work on her and I felt a need to prove myself in front of all those people."

"You did?" I was touched by his vulnerable honesty.

"Yes," said Dr. Naram, "but it only lasted for a moment. Then I did two things that my master taught me, which brought me back to my center."

"What do you mean? What did you do?"

"First, my master taught me how to bring my mind to the place

"What is the secret to coming back to your center? Silence, stillness, and solitude."

–Dr. Naram

of silence, stillness, and solitude. This returns me to the center of who I am, and when I act from that place, the results are much better. In that place, I have nothing to fear or prove, and I see that it is actually not about me at all. It is about serving the God inside the person before me. Whenever I feel off-center or don't know what to do, I go back to my center: silence, stillness, and solitude."

I didn't get it. It was as if he was speaking a foreign language. It would take me years to understand what he meant, through my own experience. At that moment, however, I simply hoped the next thing he shared would make more sense.

"What was the second thing your master taught you to do?"

Secret for Succeeding in Anything

Dr. Naram continued, "I cleaned the bathroom in a rush, eager to begin to learn pulse healing. When I came back to announce that I was done, Baba Ramdas looked surprised.

"He said, 'Let me check.'

'What do you want to check?'

'I want to check your work.'"

Dr. Naram felt self-conscious as his master inspected the bathroom. "Very bad job, Dr. Naram," Baba Ramdas said. "If you do not know how to clean the bathroom, how are you going to clean the toxins, the blocks, in people's bodies, minds, emotions, and souls?"

Dr. Naram paused, looked at me, and said, "From this experience, my master taught me this great secret: whatever you do in your life—whether it is cleaning the bathroom, preparing food, or checking the patient—do it 100 percent!"

I asked him, "But aren't there people who give 100 percent and still don't succeed?"

"That may be true, but most people do not actually give 100 percent, because they are lazy or afraid of failing. When you start to actually give 100 percent in everything you do, a different quality of enjoyment comes into your life, fear lessens, and you start to see very different results."

As Dr. Naram spoke, my mind wandered again.

If I was being honest with myself, did I give 100 percent in everything I did?

Did I even give 100 percent in anything I did?

Did I give my full effort regardless of who was watching or how important it seemed?

Unfortunately, I could think of many examples where the answer was 'no,' either because I didn't value something enough or because I had too many things going on at once. I often hid behind a computer or phone and was easily distracted from being present with people who were in the same room as me.

Dr. Naram continued, "According to my master, we cannot control other people's choices or even the results of our own choices; we can only allow those to unfold."

"But we can control our choices," I said, trying to complete his thought, "and give 100 percent in everything we do."

Secret to Success #1:
"Whatever you do in life,
give your 100 percent"
(even if it is cleaning
the toilets).

–Dr. Naram

"You got it!" he said with pleasure as I understood the first secret of the ancient teachings.

As Dr. Naram spoke, I realized he was addressing me with the same enthusiasm and intensity he does when speaking to a room of a thousand people. He was giving 100 percent in sharing this story with me, and his example impressed me more deeply than his words.

"But how do I do that—when my attention is spread among so many things?"

"Would you like me to show you a marmaa point to help you be more peaceful, present, and focused?"

"Yes, please."

He demonstrated the point he presses in order to feel more calm and present so he can give 100 percent to each person in each moment.

My Journal Notes

Marmaa Shakti Secret for Being More Peaceful, Present, and Focused*

Throughout the day, with the index finger of your right hand press the point between and just above your eyebrows 6 times.

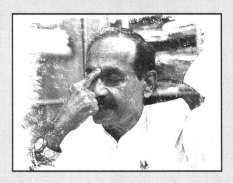

Dr. Naram said, "You asked at the beginning, how did I learn these secrets for deeper healing? Well, the simple answer is that I followed my master's words more than thirty years ago. My master told me to give 100 percent in everything I do, so I went back again right away and I cleaned that toilet with my 100 percent. When I came out, I said, 'OK, now I want to start learning,' to which my master replied, 'Your training has already begun.'"

Staying Young at Any Age

Dr. Naram studied the art and science of Siddha-Veda with his master for a thousand days. He learned secrets that were lost to the world but kept alive by an unbroken lineage of masters. Dr. Naram decided to spend the rest of his life devoted to three subjects:

1) pulse healing diagnosis and the six keys for deeper healing;
2) the secrets to living for more than a hundred years with vibrant health; and
3) the "ancient achievement system" of helping people discover, achieve, and enjoy what they want most.

Above all, Dr. Naram wanted to understand how it was possible for Baba Ramdas to be so youthful.

"Believe it or not, in my country when you are fifty-five or sixty years old, you start to think of retirement," he said. "When you are sixty, you retire and you have little enthusiasm for life. When you are sixty-five, you find yourself standing in a queue, waiting for death.

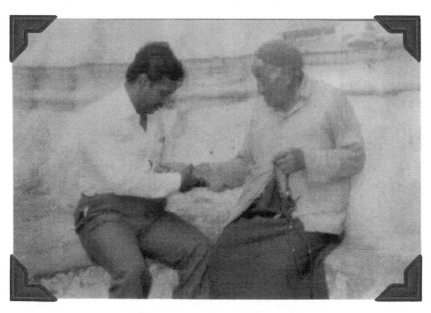

A young Dr. Naram being tested on pulse healing
by his beloved master Baba Ramdas.

Secret to Success #2:
"Make your work like a prayer. Doing work you love keeps you feeling young, no matter your age."
–Dr. Naram

This man was so different. He was 115 and had such enthusiasm for living, something I had not seen before!"

The way Dr. Naram described it was funny—people waiting in line for death. Yet his statement resonated. Many of the people I knew developed serious health problems in their fifties, sixties, and seventies. I assumed this was the way life was: you get old, your body starts to hurt and break down, then you die.

Dr. Naram said, "When people would ask my master, 'How old are you?' he would say, 'I am 115 years *young*, and many years to go.' And at the same time, he was healthy, alert, and still working hard."

As that settled in, I marveled at what a different expectation Dr. Naram had about life from seeing his master feel 'young' at 115 years.

"Can I share with you another million-dollar secret?"

"Yes."

"Whereas in many countries people try to retire and get out of work, in my lineage we are lovers of work. For us, work is like prayer. Doing work you love keeps you feeling young, no matter your age."

"How did your master do it?" I asked. "What was his secret for being young at any age?"

"Now you are asking a billion-dollar question. Just be prepared, if I teach this to you, it will change your life forever."

"OK." I became even more alert, opening my notebook to a new page.

"From sharing only parts of this secret now with thousands and thousands of people from all over the world, from 108 countries, results come which they call 'miracles.' After trying so many other things that didn't work, when they try even part of this secret, they often experience deeper healing. Their diabetes reduces or goes away. Their arthritis pain subsides, and they can start to walk again. Or their frozen shoulder gets unstuck, their child with ADD or ADHD improves, their hair grows back if they were bald, their sleep improves, they lose weight, their depression lessens, their allergies and asthma go away, their skin gets better, their energy and stamina increase, and so many other things.

"It is not only the secret behind how my master lived to such old age, but also how he continued to have so much flexibility, mental power, enthusiasm, and vibrant health."

"What did he do?" I asked. "Can you share it with me?"

Dr. Naram hesitated for a moment, then leaned toward me and said in a hushed but energetic voice: "Siddha-Veda has six secret keys of deeper healing, which can transform anyone's body, mind, and emotions—the six keys by which you have now seen 'impossible' situations become possible."

There was the sound of a honking horn. He stopped and looked outside the window. There was our taxi, to take Alicia and me to the airport. I asked quickly, "What are they? What are the six keys of deeper healing? How can I learn them?"

"Come tomorrow," he said with a twinkle in his eye.

"But I can't. I'm going to New York and then on to Utah."

He smiled, paused again, then slowly said, "For some reason God has brought you to me, and me to you, don't you think?"

I nodded, and he continued, "The next time we meet, if we meet again, perhaps I will share with you these six powerful keys that my master shared with me, the lost ancient secret for staying young at any age."

We proceeded outside, where Alicia was already waiting by the taxi. As I opened the car door to get in, Dr. Naram called to me and said, "It would be very good if you could meet with Marianjii in New York."

> *"Siddha-Veda has six secret keys of deeper healing, which can transform anyone's body, mind, and emotions."*
>
> –Dr. Naram

Your Journal Notes

To deepen and magnify the benefits you will experience from reading this book, take a few minutes now and answer the following questions for yourself:

How do you feel ego and fear impact your life?

_____

_____

_____

_____

_____

How do you feel your life might change for the better if you were less impacted by fear and ego?

_____

_____

_____

_____

_____

What other insights, questions, or realizations came to you as you read this chapter?

_____

_____

_____

_____

_____

CHAPTER 6

Can Cow's Ghee & Secret Points on Your Body Bring Your Blood Pressure to Normal in Minutes?

Reason is powerless in the expression of love. Your task is not to seek for love, but merely to seek and find all the barriers within yourself that you have built against it.

–Rumi

New York City

Parting with Alicia at the airport in Mumbai was bittersweet. Although disappointed that we weren't headed into a relationship, I was pleased she was happy with what she experienced in India and had a clearer vision of where she wanted to take her life.

Anxious as I was to reach my father, I was glad I had an eighteen-hour layover in New York. That would give me enough time to see some of the sights and meet with Marianjii, who was with Dr. Naram that first day I met him in LA. Perhaps she could help answer some of my questions.

Before landing at JFK Airport, I had seen New York City only in TV shows and movies. The weather was clear and cool, the opposite of Mumbai, and I was glad I brought a coat and gloves. I took the subway to Times Square, recognizing from television the spot where the ball drops on New Year's Eve, surrounded on every side by the flashing lights of jumbo screens advertising products and Broadway shows. I passed thousands of people in the streets, speaking dozens of different languages, all gazing at the screens and storefronts.

As I walked the streets, I felt like an ant, made tiny by the endless wall of skyscrapers. People, sights, sounds, and smells filled the streets. Only when I arrived at Central Park did the buildings give way to greenery. I bought some hot nuts from a street vendor, loving his New York accent.

I walked to the famous Macy's store, which I recognized from when I was a kid watching the Thanksgiving Day Parade on TV, and from our family watching and rewatching *Miracle on 34th Street*. Stepping inside the Borders bookstore attached to Madison Square Garden, I warmed up with a hot drink and wandered among the shelves and tables displaying hundreds of books. My eyes were drawn to one I'd not heard of before with a title I didn't understand—*The Alchemist*. I bought it without knowing why.

By early afternoon I had seen the Empire State Building, Fifth Avenue, the Chrysler Building, the Rockefeller Center, the Brooklyn Bridge, the UN headquarters, the Metropolitan Museum of Art, and a bustling Wall Street. I was amazed by how much I saw of New York City in one day alone, and by how much more there was left to see.

Then I had a moment to pause. An eerie feeling came over me as I approached the site of the former World Trade Center Twin Towers, which fell during the terrorist attacks on September 11, 2001. Looking through the fence, I saw gaping holes in the ground where the buildings once stood. Although the rubble had been removed and the site was being built into a memorial, I felt echoes of the devastation. Everyone I know who was alive at that time remembers where they were when they heard about the planes crashing into those buildings. We all watched on the news the towers going up in flames and tumbling to the ground as people scrambled to get away, covered in dust. I was at my youngest sister's apartment when she said, "Did you hear? New York is under attack!" We watched smoke coming from the first tower as a plane crashed into the second. Horrified, I wondered who was attacking us, why, and how could I protect myself and my family.

On that day, 2,977 people from 115 different nations died there, including 441 emergency workers who responded to the call to help; among them were firefighters, paramedics, police officers, and emergency medical technicians. I was shocked to learn that many more people died in the aftermath of the attack due to the toxins they were exposed to.

Leaving this somber memorial site, I walked to Battery Park. I spotted something completely familiar, though I'd never seen it in person before—the Statue of Liberty. Looking at the iconic lady holding her book and torch, I thought about the many different things the United States represented to people all over the world. What did it mean to my friends in Europe, to the people in India I just met, to the Native Americans who were here long before the immigrants, and to the terrorists who plummeted those planes into the Twin Towers?

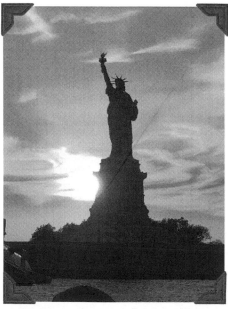

The Statue of Liberty on Liberty Island
in New York.

Deep in thought, my senses overwhelmed, I arrived at Grand Central Station and boarded the train to Westchester County. As the train idled at station after station, I saw a part of New York rarely depicted in movies. Once we left the skyscrapers behind, there was endless green surrounding beautiful lakes and rivers, interspersed with small towns and cities. Finally, in a moment of peace and solitude, my mind turned toward my upcoming meeting with Marianjii.

He Saved My Life

Marianjii was born in Iran to a Russian father and a Persian mother. She was now living in New York and had been helping Dr. Naram for several years. I was nervous about meeting with her in her home. She had a strong and direct personality, and although we had met once before, I worried that she wouldn't like me.

As if she could read my unspoken feelings, when I arrived, out of the blue, Marianjii told me that it wasn't her concern whether people liked her or not. "It would be very small of me if I only helped those I like or who like me," she said.

To mitigate my discomfort, I began to ask questions. Over moong bean soup, she told me about her life. Marianjii credited Dr. Naram with saving her life on more than one occasion, including once during a trip overseas.

"During the trip, Dr. Naram asked me, 'Is your blood pressure high?' I responded, 'No, my blood pressure is always low.'"

"When I was a child," she told me, "my mother suffered a severe stroke. She was completely paralyzed and couldn't even close her eyes to sleep; they had to cover them with a dark piece of cloth so she could rest. I had thought she was invincible and had all the answers, and now seeing her lying there so vulnerable, I felt so sad, small, and helpless."

As Marianjii spoke, I thought of my own mother. Despite our challenges, she always seemed so strong to me, almost unstoppable. *What would it be like if one day I found my mom immobilized and powerless? What would I do?* I was glad when Marianjii continued talking—I wanted to shake that thought from my head.

"I did not want people to see me crying," Marianjii said, "so I hid behind the curtains. I was so confused, I kept turning and spinning as the curtains bunched and snagged my hair. The pain of my hair being pulled was the only sensation I could feel—almost sobering, bringing a sense of presence to the otherwise numbing experience. My mother was only thirty-nine. She was crippled and paralyzed on her right side for the rest of her life after that. From that moment on, I always remembered that what hurt my mother was high blood pressure."

> *"It would be very small of me if I only helped those I like or who like me."*
>
> –Marianjii

Since high blood pressure led to her mother's stroke, Marianjii feared hypertension, so she had her blood pressure measured often.

Four hours before flying home, Dr. Naram asked again if she had high blood pressure. Marianjii was so certain her blood pressure was fine that she asked him to check it in order to put his mind at ease. She was shocked to find out that it was extremely high—220/118! It could easily cause a stroke or worse. Getting on a seventeen-hour flight was out of the question.

"Dr. Naram looked at me seriously and asked if I would allow him to help me. My fear and the memories of my mother's struggle and suffering flooded my brain. I was so overwhelmed and anxious. I couldn't calm down."

Dr. Naram told her to lie down with her head on a pillow. He applied one finger-scoop of ghee to the very top of her head, lightly tapping, allowing the ghee to penetrate into her skull. Then he applied another finger-scoop of ghee to each temple simultaneously, moving his fingers in a clockwise circular motion. Next, he placed one scoop of ghee in her navel, then on the arch of each foot. He did the entire process twice.

"At this point, Dr. Naram rechecked my blood pressure," Marianjii said. "It had dropped almost forty points, now registering at 182/104. Dr. Naram repeated the process once more, and my blood pressure dropped again to 168/94. He was not yet comfortable with the results, knowing I had to endure a long journey back to New York. He repeated the process once again, and afterward I was close to my normal blood pressure, 120/75."

"Wow, that is incredible," I said.

"I know it may seem simple or even primitive to some," she said, "but ancient healing can be extremely effective. And it's not just for emergencies. Marmaa, in addition to the other keys of Siddha-Veda, can be done regularly for long-term results. Thanks to these secrets, I have maintained normal blood pressure for nearly seven years without the help of any medication."

My Journal Notes

Ancient Healing Secrets for Maintaining Normal Blood Pressure*

1) Marmaa Shakti—Put a scoop of ghee on top of head, in navel, and on the bottom of feet. Also rub ghee in a circular motion on the temples of your forehead, pressing downward on the last motion. Take a few deep breaths, rest for five to ten minutes, then begin the process again.

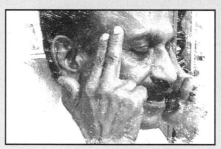

2) Herbal Remedies—She took an herbal formula created for supporting healthy blood pressure, which included ingredients like arjuna bark and Indian pennywort; and one herbal formula for calming the mind, which included ingredients like water hyssop, gotu kola, licorice, and ashwaganda.*

*Information (including key ingredients) for herbal formulas mentioned in this book are in the appendix. Bonus Material: To see this marmaa demonstrated, please refer to the free membership site.

"Can you tell me more about where Siddha-Veda came from?"

"The ancient healing art and science of Siddha-Veda is among the oldest and most intricate recorded forms of medicine. The ancient texts containing healing techniques and instructions have been passed on from the master healers to chosen students for generations. The masters' nomadic existence played an important role in gathering information. Traveling doctors are exposed to different environments, illnesses, and cultures. They also learn from locals about their healing methods and regional medicinal herbs.

"The ancient manuscripts were handed down to Dr. Naram by his master, Baba Ramdas, who at that time was the head of the lineage. He lived to 125 years, and before passing on to the next life, he bestowed the head of the lineage to Dr. Naram. Along with the manuscripts, Dr. Naram was given the title of *Siddha Nadi Vaidya*, meaning 'Master of Pulse Healing.'

"The way Dr. Naram brought my blood pressure down in less than an hour without medication is something that most modern doctors do not understand, but anyone who wants to learn this method can easily do so and benefit from it."

Serving Those Who Serve

Two visitors came to Marianjii's home the same day I arrived: Marshall Stackman and José Mestre. They were the co-founders (along with Rosemary Nulty and Nechemiah Bar-Yehuda) of a nonprofit organization called Serving Those Who Serve (STWS). Together they led an effort to help firefighters, police officers, and other first responders affected by 9/11. It turned out to be one of those meetings I wished could have lasted longer.

"After the dust settled, most people went back to their lives," Marshall explained. "But more than thirty thousand first responders inhaled toxic fumes or absorbed them through their skin, which affected their lungs, their digestion, their sleep, and their minds, making life much more difficult."

José said, "It was my connection with Dr. Naram that gave me the idea that perhaps ancient healing could help where other methods proved insufficient. I attended a workshop with Dr. Naram earlier, which gave me clarity on what I wanted to do with my life. I knew I wanted to help these firefighters and first responders." He shared how these brave people suffered from a variety of conditions, such as depression, pulmonary issues, PTSD, black spots on their lungs, and memory loss, just to name a few. Marshall and José were proud to show me a stack of written accounts from firefighters and others who benefited from the herbal supplements of Dr. Naram, provided at no cost to them.

They told me about Virginia Brown, a former NYPD officer who worked for eight months at Ground Zero while debris was still being cleared away. She was helping in a trauma unit and supporting security, and despite wearing a mask most of the time, she developed a persistent cough. Her lung capacity decreased, the toxins affected her bones and joints, and she couldn't sleep well. One of the medical workers told her about the STWS program and she did not hesitate. After she took the herbs for two years, her doctor was stunned.

They showed me a letter she'd written: "There are a lot of police officers and other workers from Ground Zero with similar problems that have gotten worse. Many died. I know some who contracted cancer, emphysema, and problems from different lung ailments that wouldn't go away. But my lung capacity was improving. The doctor was amazed. My bones also improved instead of getting worse! I really believe it has a lot to do with Dr. Naram's herbal formulas, because those I know who didn't take them just got worse. Even after retiring, I still take the herbs, and overall, I feel they contribute in a positive way to my health. I'm sleeping much better and my whole body regulates better. Thanks so much for all of it."

As I listened, I thought the story was beautiful, and because of things I had already seen, part of me wanted to believe it was all true. At the same time, I realized stories like this one are only anecdotal, and I wanted more evidence. Perhaps she got better for other reasons. I asked, "Is there solid evidence proving that it was the herbs that helped her? Surely the government must have provided the best medical care possible to the heroes of 9/11. Couldn't it be that something else she was taking is actually what helped her?"

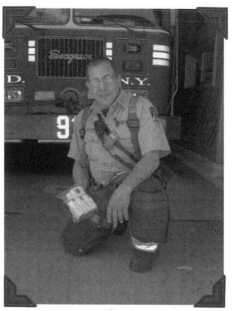

FDNY Firefighter who benefited from the herbal formulas.

"There was no lack of care or help given to these people," José said. "Medical doctors showed up from everywhere to lend support. They gave their best efforts, but people still suffered. When other methods were insufficient to help them, the herbs from Dr. Naram worked wonders."

"But don't take our word for it," Marshall said. He handed me a peer-reviewed article published in a medical journal (*Alternative Therapies in Health and Medicine*) that documented a study of the 9/11 first responders who participated in the pilot program sponsored by STWS. "The study was conducted by two highly respected physicians, who documented the experiences of firefighters and other first responders who used Dr. Naram's herbal formulas versus conventional medical treatments."

According to researchers, those taking the herbs experienced "significant improvements." They said the results seen in "this high-risk, toxin-exposed population" were especially noticed "for specific symptoms that had been reported as not improving under conventional medical treatment, including cough, difficulty breathing, fatigue, exhaustion, not feeling well, difficulty sleeping, and other symptoms." The report described a lack of negative side effects from the herbs, other than a small percent who had slight gastric discomfort for a few days when starting. The participants in the study saw significant improvement with previously unresolved medical symptoms; they no longer needed inhalers, their sleep improved greatly, immunity improved, coughing stopped, cysts disappeared, black spots on their lungs vanished, memory improved, depression and fatigue decreased, their energy was boosted, and they had hope again.

"We have so many stories like this I can share with you," said Marshall. "Ninety-eight percent of participants in the study said they would recommend the herbal program to a friend with similar symptoms. And they did, which is why the program is growing, and why we came to talk with Marianjii. We need to figure out how to get more herbs and get them regularly."

"Usually, there is crisis in a developing country," José added, "like people starving in India or Africa, and the United States or Europe helps. This is one of the first examples that I know of where someone from a so-called developing country is coming to a world power like the United States and doing such great humanitarian work. Dr. Naram helped, and continues to help, people in the United States during our crisis in a way we desperately need, and at his own expense!"

I wanted to hear more, but there was a honking horn outside. Once again, a taxi was waiting to take me to an airport.

Marianjii walked me to the door. Looking straight into my eyes, she said, "I have a feeling there is a reason you were led to this. Perhaps there is a relationship that existed even before your birth. Who knows, maybe we were led to you because of something you are meant to do in your life, and in ours."

Unsure of how to respond, I thanked her for her time and got into the taxi. As I looked out the back window to her house, I noticed the difference in how I was feeling now versus when I came. I had a lot to think about. The way Marianjii, Marshall, and

José spoke about Dr. Naram and his work, with so much candid conviction, made me question my own skepticism. My encounter with them made me reflect on my beliefs about things like what foods were good for me, how long it was possible for someone to live, and why I was alive now. Maybe my beliefs were limited, based on misinformation. And maybe they were holding me back from something better.

> *"I have a feeling there is a reason you were led to this."*
>
> –Marianjii

Seeing these methods work on other people was remarkable, but I had reservations. I still thought the success of Dr. Naram's treatment was due to the placebo effect. Or perhaps coming from a trick that was available only to Dr. Naram. I wanted to learn more.

Your Journal Notes

To deepen and magnify the benefits you will experience from reading this book, take a few minutes now and answer the following questions for yourself:

What have you been exposed to that has been physically, mentally, and/or emotionally toxic?

_____

_____

_____

_____

_____

Why do you feel you were led to this book about ancient healing?

_____

_____

_____

_____

_____

What other insights, questions, or realizations came to you as you read this chapter?

_____

_____

_____

_____

CHAPTER 7

A Moment That Changed My Life

The place you are right now, God circled on a map for you.

–Hafiz

Utah

When I reached my parents' home in Midvale, Utah, my dad greeted me at the door. I inhaled the aroma of homemade bread my mom had just taken out of the oven. She warmly greeted me from the kitchen before getting back to the many tasks on her to-do list. I could tell both she and my dad were relieved I was there. As I looked into my dad's eyes, I noticed that beneath his gentle smile was deep concern, and heading toward his office I saw physical discomfort in the way he walked.

As he closed the door behind us, I sat in the chair in front of his desk, and he sat in one off to the side. There was a long silence as he looked at the ground. He seemed to be considering how to start.

His eyes slowly moved up to meet my confused gaze.

"I haven't told your mother," he began, "and I haven't told your brothers or sisters yet." There was a long pause as his eyes dropped to the ground again. His brow furrowed, and his face tightened with a deep consternation. My eyes widened with worry and the uncertainty that gripped me. He lifted his gaze from the floor, making eye contact with me only for a split-second before quickly shifting his gaze to the empty space beside me. He raised his right hand to his forehead, slowly rubbing it with his fingers. Although his hand partially covered his face from me, I saw his eyes fill with water. Struggling to get the words out, he finally said, "I don't even know if I'm going to live through this week."

My mouth was open, but I was silent with shock as I watched him rub the tears from his eyes. *Had I heard him correctly?* This caught me completely off guard. It felt like someone sucker-punched me in the gut. My head was spinning. Whatever else was on my mind before this meeting suddenly faded into the distance of complete insignificance. My heart pounded. *I couldn't lose my father. I wasn't ready. Not this soon. Not like this.* I needed to know more.

"What's happening, Dad?"

"I don't know how to tell you this." He struggled telling me as much as I struggled listening. "There is so much pain in my entire body that it feels like someone has slammed me against the wall. At night I lie awake in so much agony that..." Again his brow furrowed and his face tightened as his gaze dropped down at the ground.

"What, Dad?"

With his eyes still on the ground, and shaking his head side to side slowly he said, "I know that no son should ever have to hear this from his father, but when I'm in this much pain I honestly don't know if I even want to live to see the morning."

His words sank in my heart like boulders. My dad was always a positive person. He'd rarely talk about his challenges, and if he ever did, he always put a twist of optimism to it—that things were getting better, or that he had good people helping him. I never heard him utter a sentence as bleak as this before. And I couldn't control my feelings.

My dad looked up as I wiped away the fresh tears pouring down my cheeks. He reached up and gently put his right hand on my shoulder.

Losing my sister as a child had such an impact, I couldn't handle losing my dad, too. I always assumed he would be at my future wedding and read stories to my future kids. There were so many questions I never asked him and things I never did with him because I assumed there would be time. Was it possible that now I only had a few precious days left with him?

With my mind going wild, I tried to bring my focus back to what was most important in this moment. I pulled myself together long enough to ask, "How can I help you, Dad?"

"Yes, I do need your help, Son," he said. "You've always been responsible, and I need to let someone know where my records, accounts, and passwords are. In case I'm not alive one morning, I don't want any confusion or loose ends for your mother to have to deal with."

He spoke deliberately, maintaining his composure, but it was clear he was exhausted and depressed. As he opened the drawer of his desk to pull out the folder with his passwords, I noticed something else behind it. Normally on top of his desk was a stack of papers. He gathered them for his dream of writing a book to encompass his life's work. Now they were set aside, tucked out of the way in the desk. A shoe-box filled with bottles of various medications stood now in their place.

"Son, at this point you are the only one I'm saying anything to because I don't want the others to worry, but I need to set everything in order."

I didn't want to accept what he was saying about his life ending, but I knew that taking down his passwords would give him peace of mind. I listened as best as I could.

Then I began to question him again. "What treatments are you on? There must be something else we can do that would help!"

"I'm visiting four highly qualified doctors, who are trying everything they can think of. Two of the four specialists told me just this month that they didn't know what else they could do for me. They said they tried everything they know of and have now run out of ideas. The other two don't have much hope either."

My dad had been suffering for years, but because he never complained, we had no idea it was this bad. He was seventy-one, but when he was twenty-five, he was diagnosed with rheumatoid arthritis, for which he'd been given strong medications. The side effects caused other serious problems, and he was sent to other doctors and prescribed more medications. Now he was on twelve medications for a litany of things, including high cholesterol, high blood pressure, chest pain, leg pain, diabetes, sleeping problems, gastrointestinal problems, unbearable arthritis pain, low energy, increasing depression, and a fading memory from the onset of early dementia. His own mother had severe Alzheimer's and he feared it was coming on strong for him, too. On top of that, he had two stents in his heart, and there'd been talk of bypass surgery.

In the absence of any other solution, and amidst a feeling of desperation, I said: "Dad, I haven't told you much about my trip to India. Can I share more about what I witnessed there?"

I hadn't said much before because I didn't know how to make sense of it myself. But now I told my dad all the stories I could remember, of things that might bring him hope that healing was possible.

"Also, Dad, for Father's Day I want to give you something," I said, taking a deep breath. "I want to buy you a plane ticket to see Dr. Naram, wherever he is traveling next."

I thought the possibility of meeting Dr. Naram would bring my dad hope, but instead he looked more exhausted. With so much pain in his body, just the thought of flying drained him. But more than that, he couldn't imagine that simply by touching his pulse, anyone could help him. Especially when extensive medical testing and care from the best doctors could not.

"I've already tried alternative therapies," he said. "I tried homeopathy, reflexology, acupuncture, Chinese medicine, and more. They all promised great results, but in my case never delivered much relief. Really, Son, I just want you to remember where my passwords are."

"Dad, just trust me on this. Can we at least try?" The tension I felt must have been evident in the intensity of my request.

"At this point," he said, forcing a smile, "the good news is, at least I have nothing to lose."

California
Back in the City of Angels

The truth was, I didn't know if Dr. Naram could help my dad, but I had nowhere else to turn. I went online, found Dr. Naram's schedule, called the phone number, and booked an appointment for my dad at the location in LA. I wasted no time.

When we arrived, there was already a crowd of people waiting. Several dozen people were filling out paperwork or waiting for their names to be called. My dad looked tired and pale from the travel and the pain in his body. The wait time, I was told, was anywhere between three to six hours.

There were even more people than usual because of an event Dr. Naram spoke at the day before. I was surprised to hear from others that while he was on the stage, he received a six-minute standing ovation. While my dad and I waited, every once in a while someone would come out of their consultation with Dr. Naram and approach me.

They would ask, "Are you Dr. Clint?"

"Yes, but I'm not a medical doctor. I'm a university researcher," I clarified.

"Dr. Naram asked me to share my story with you."

I'd ask their name and we'd talk about what brought them to Dr. Naram. I was surprised again by how far people traveled to see him, coming from all around the world. I noticed how they were remarkably diverse, people of almost every race, ethnicity, religion, and socioeconomic status.

My dad looked too tired to engage in the conversations, so I took them to the side of the room or hallway to talk. Between conversations, I went back to my dad to share what I learned.

A first-time patient revealed how Dr. Naram described everything that was wrong with her without her saying a word. This included identifying problems with two of her vertebrae. She showed me medical reports and scans that confirmed what he identified in her pulse. Another man was amazed how Dr. Naram knew about his diabetes and heart blockage just from feeling his pulse. Dr. Naram correctly predicted, within one-tenth of a point, what his blood sugar level was and accurately described how blocked his artery was. A hotel owner from the area told me he had severe celiac disease. Before seeing Dr. Naram, eating food with any gluten caused him unbelievable pain. "Now I can eat an entire pizza and drink a couple of beers with no problem."

I was curious what caused all these people—the Americans in particular—to be open to this alternative healing method. I asked Dr. Giovanni, who I knew had trained with Dr. Naram in India for some time. He challenged my phrasing and said he didn't know why Dr. Naram's approach was called "alternative," as it was thousands of years older than Western medicine. He said, if anything, what Dr. Naram and other traditional healers were doing should be considered the original, and Western medicine should be the alternative. He preferred the term "complementary healing," as these modalities do not need to be in conflict.

While speaking to Dr. Giovanni, I saw my dad shifting in his chair in obvious discomfort.

Upon hearing this physician's confidence in Dr. Naram's method, I confided in him something that was troubling me. "I know for most people, Dr. Naram describes accurately what they are feeling from touching their pulse. But I've also talked with others who said he missed something important when he took their pulse, and they felt disappointed."

"How many people have you talked with, total?" he asked me.

"So far, between India and here, probably about a hundred."

"And of those people, how many said he missed something?"

After reflecting, I replied, "maybe two or three."

"First, isn't it remarkable that his average is so high? According to your sample size, that is ninety-seven percent accuracy. That is also in a short period of time and with such a wide variety of issues. Do you know that in Western medicine, even after extensive testing we doctors often can't identify the source of the problem? For example, we can see there is high blood pressure by measuring it, but only about 20 percent of the time we can identify the cause. That means 80 percent of the time we just make our best guess and prescribe medications to control it. If the medications cause too many side effects, then we test out another medication to see if it works better. I'm not saying Dr. Naram is perfect or doesn't make mistakes. Remarkably capable as he is, he is still human. I'm just recognizing that the percentage of times he succeeds in correctly identifying the core problem and helping people heal from it when they follow his advice is extremely high.

"How can ancient healing be called 'alternative,' as it is thousands of years older than Western medicine? If anything, it could be called 'complementary healing,' as these modalities do not need to be in conflict at all."

–Dr. Giovanni

"And one other thing you should know is that Dr. Naram uses a different paradigm and vocabulary for describing problems than Western medicine does. He has an ancient method of understanding and classifying illnesses and what he would call 'dis-ease' instead of disease. A few people over the years have also asked me why he missed something in their pulse. When I went back to look at Dr. Naram's notes, I saw that he actually identified the core problem correctly according to the lens of his ancient healing science, even if he didn't name the disease according to the Western lexicon. For example, in his lineage, they don't have a problem called cancer. They don't see cancer as the problem. What we call cancer, they see as a symptom of a deeper imbalance they call *tri-doshar*. And these master healers utilize sophisticated, time-tested methods for resolving that imbalance, with extensive experience showing that it and its symptoms can then slowly disappear."

I didn't fully understand what he said, so I asked more questions. But more than his answers, it was his confidence that eased some of my concern. I was searching for as many assurances as possible that I wasn't crazy to bring my dad here. Each time I walked back to sit next to my dad, he forced a smile before going back to shifting in his chair. This time, I brought him some water. Weakly holding the cup with both hands, he gratefully drank it.

Several more patients came up to me who were born in places like India, Pakistan, and Bangladesh but who now lived in the United States. In addition to hearing their experience with Dr. Naram, I learned a lot more about what their lives were like. One mother told me, "My husband and I came to America hoping it would benefit our children. Only it broke my heart when my children lost interest in our Indian culture, faith, and traditions. Instead, they became addicted to their phones and computers and more interested in their friends than in school." She worried her children would break tradition and not take care of her and her husband in old age.

There was a group of young people from India and Pakistan now studying and working in California. One thing or another eventually led them to Dr. Naram for help.

"Kids like us often struggle with our identity," one young man told me, "not feeling like we belong to either culture." Even when they got into the best universities in America, some were attracted to drugs, alcohol, sex, and relationships with people their parents didn't approve of. This made them feel distant from their families. "We often struggle to find a decent job, being kept in lower positions and expected to work harder for less pay and less respect because of our residential status." I was sad to hear that sometimes young women were asked for sexual favors by their employers, simply to keep the job that allowed them to stay in the country.

One female student said, "I'm stressed because of school and relationships, and eat food that's not good for me. I was diagnosed with hormonal imbalance and gained lots of weight. Then I got acne and other skin problems. A few years ago, I was a model for magazines, and now I don't even want to go out. I don't feel good about myself, and I worry I'll never get married like this. In my frustration, I've started resenting my parents and heritage for the pressure on me to be perfect when I'm not perfect." Her words affected me. I also felt pressure to be perfect when I knew I was not.

Then the story of one young lawyer inspired me. His parents were from India. They moved to the United States when he was young, so he didn't feel a strong connection to India. In some ways, he actually looked down on his parents' culture. "Then, while I was in law school," he said, "I developed a problem called vitiligo, which causes white patches to grow on your skin. It spread on my arms first, then to my hands and face. Many young people with this condition struggle with self-esteem and worry it will affect their marriageability. There were no Western treatments that offered a cure. So it seemed improbable to me that Dr. Naram could help."

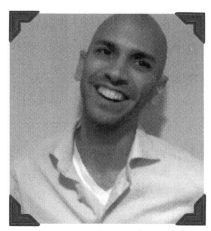

Samir, a young lawyer from Boston who overcame vitiligo.

But Samir tried anyway. "Slowly at first the color started coming back, and two years later all the white spots were gone! There are lots of Indian Americans like me who've grown up mostly in America and who don't have much respect for our Indian culture. Dr. Naram's methods," he said, "have changed me in more ways than one. If I had not taken the time to experience it myself, I wouldn't have believed in it." Seeing that the solution to this problem wasn't found anywhere in Western medicine, but came from an Indian specialist of the ancient healing science, he said, "I gained more respect for my culture, my heritage, and where I'm from than I otherwise would have."

"If I had not taken the time to experience it myself, I wouldn't have believed in ancient healing. But it has given me more respect for my culture, my heritage, and where I am from than I otherwise would have had."

–Samir

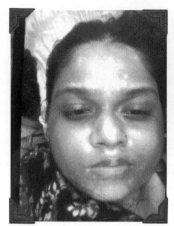 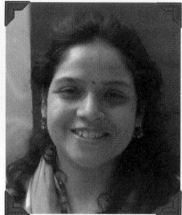

Left: Woman with vitiligo for 10 years. Right: Months after discipline with Dr. Naram's diet and herbs.

My Journal Notes

Three Ancient Healing Secrets for Great Skin*

1) Marmaa Shakti—On both sides of the top knuckle of the right hand ring finger, press and release 6 times, many times a day.

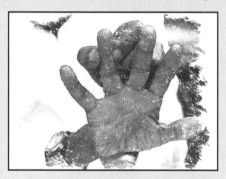

2) Herbal Remedies—Samir used a cream and took some herbal tablets for skin, which included ingredients like neem, turmeric, coconut oil, holy basil, and black pepper.*

3) Diet Secrets—Eat only foods that are gluten-free, dairy-free, and sugar-free.

*Information (including key ingredients) for herbal formulas mentioned in this book are in the appendix. Bonus Material: To discover more secrets for great skin, please visit the free MyAncientSecrets.com membership site.

A beautiful young Muslim couple walked up to me next. "We left our home country to live in America, with the hope of more peace and opportunity," the husband told me. "Then we arrived here only to find that many people treated us poorly, fearing we were terrorists. We worked hard to make new friends and show that true Islam is about peace. We came to America hoping to have a family and raise kids, but that dream was shattered." Doctors diagnosed the young man with azoospermia, which meant his sperm count was zero.

"We tried for six years," he told me. "We went to so many specialists and spent nearly eighty thousand dollars on all kinds of other ways to have a baby, but Western medicine had no solution for us. It was draining us financially and emotionally. We were devastated. Then we met Dr. Naram. We followed everything exactly as he told us to do for deeper healing, and within a year, I went back to be tested and my sperm count was five million. The doctors said it was a miracle, questioning whether the first test had been right." He showed me the medical reports from before and after. "Within two years, my wife was pregnant," his voice cracked with emotion as he spoke, "and today we came just to show Dr. Naram our baby and say thank you." Noticing the tears coming down his wife's cheeks, he reached out to hug her and rub her back gently, both looking at their 'miracle' baby together.

A Sikh man by the name of Gurcharan Singh, wearing a turban and a long beard, joined me. He told me he was involved in politics in Bakersfield, California. I learned that Sikhs are some of the most misunderstood people in America. This man felt strongly that Dr. Naram understood them. "Dr. Naram has helped me, my family, and my friends overcome so many challenges like high cholesterol, arthritis, diabetes, high blood pressure, and hormonal imbalance." Out of gratitude, he arranged for the mayor of Bakersfield, California, to give Dr. Naram an award for his support and contributions to the Sikh community. "Do you know one of Dr. Naram's patients was Yogi Bhajan Singh, maybe the most well-known Sikh in the world?" he said.

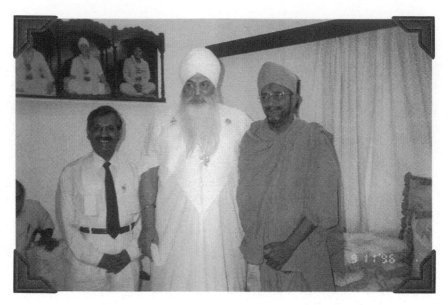

Dr. Naram with Yogi Bhajan Singh & H.H. Hariprasad Swamiji.

I was very interested in what Gurcharan and others said, because I wanted to know if Dr. Naram could indeed help my dad. When I first went to India, my skepticism was about 80 percent and my curiosity, 20 percent. I now had enough evidence that most people were getting better, but I didn't know in what proportion it produced lasting change. I also didn't know if the healing was attributed to the possibility that Dr. Naram just convinced them that they'd get better, so they did. At this point, after seeing and hearing numerous remarkable cases, I'd say that my skepticism melted to about 50 percent. While I still felt guarded, the other 50 percent was a mixture of increasing curiosity and a wild hope that what Dr. Naram did was a predictable way of healing people, or at the very least, could help my dad. Only, while I was more hopeful with each experience I heard, the pain in my dad's body was getting worse. I booked a room in the hotel and took my dad to rest there until it was closer to his turn.

A Healer in Need of Healing

When I returned to the waiting room, an older but fit-looking bearded gentleman came up to me. With a warm, firm handshake, he introduced himself as Rabbi Stephen Robbins. Besides being a rabbi and a Kabbalist—a practitioner of an ancient Jewish spiritual tradition—he was also a clinical psychologist. He was the co-founder of the Academy for Jewish Religion, California, the first transdenominational seminary on the West Coast.

Several years earlier, Stephen had several near-death experiences due to a number of illnesses. Prior to the illnesses, he was healthy and athletic, able to lift 300 pounds. Then muscular dystrophy began eating away at his muscle mass. Doctors gave him massive doses of cortisone, which caused horrible osteoporosis. On top of that, he caught influenza, his lungs collapsed twice, and he died—twice—before being resuscitated. His various health crises disrupted the function of his hypothalamus, pituitary gland, and entire endocrine system to the point that he produced no testosterone or growth hormone (HGH) on his own. Without that, his cells could not regenerate.

"I did everything I could, but nothing worked," Stephen explained. "The medications and treatments were barely holding me in place. In 2005, I got hit with another lung infection, and my lungs collapsed again."

Stephen spent weeks in the hospital before he was able to breathe independently. Just as he was getting ready to go home, he came down with a severe case of shingles, which affected the discs in his back. The shingles affected the nerves on the right side of his torso so severely that he lived in excruciating pain all the time. "I was experiencing nerve pain that felt like lightning bolts from front to back and back to front, skin pain similar to feeling acid on your skin, as well as muscle pain causing spasms that made it hard to function or breathe."

"After taking methadone and painkillers for seven months, I sounded like an idiot and felt as though I might be a vegetable for the rest of my life. The doctors didn't know what to do."

Things kept getting worse until a friend encouraged Stephen to see Dr. Naram.

"The whole concept of being able to diagnose a person in just a few moments seems irrational to the Western mind, where we are committed to the Western paradigm of blood tests, MRIs, and multiple doctors. Dr. Naram's model of healing, however, is not based on being ill, but on being well. It's a totally different approach in which your body, mind, and spirit are able to participate with you in deeper healing."

He looked me in the eye and said, "I have been a rabbi and a healer since I was sixteen years old, and now at sixty-one, meeting Dr. Naram was the first time in my life, I could just let go and surrender myself into other hands to heal me. It was a profound moment."

Wondering how his experience might relate to my father's, I listened attentively. Stephen arrived in India at Dr. Naram's clinic in a wheelchair, weak and desperate. He had to bring synthetic HGH just to stay alive, instructing his host that it needed to be refrigerated. To make matters worse, his host accidentally destroyed the entire supply by putting it in the freezer. Stephen was devastated. He called his American doctors for a solution, but there was nothing that they could do. He turned to Dr. Naram.

Dr. Naram prepared a special mixture of healing herbs, based on the principles of his ancient lineage, to regenerate HGH and restore testosterone levels.

"I had no other choice, so I followed his instructions exactly. By the end of the first week, I was out of the wheelchair, feeling stronger each day. By the third week, I took a blood test to see what was happening. And this is when I saw what I consider the miracle of miracles. After all that trauma, the new blood tests showed something remarkable. For the first time in years, my body was producing its own human growth hormone—and at levels that were equivalent to those in people much younger than me! Before, I was taking synthetic testosterone too, but now my body is producing testosterone again on its own. My thyroid is pretty much back to normal. My pancreas, thank God, is normal. My thymus and immune system are supported by the healing herbs and are functioning well.

"The healing continued, and when I got off the plane, my wife did not recognize me. I had lost thirty pounds and was stronger. She said I looked like I did when we first met, thirty years ago. My hair was darker and thicker, too. It was amazing."

Since then, the rabbi had gone back to the gym. To prove his point, he pulled his shirt sleeve up to his shoulder and flexed his now-solid bicep. I couldn't help but smile with him. The image of a delighted rabbi showing me his flexed bicep with a child-like joy in his eyes will never leave me.

Wondering how I could describe his healing experience to my dad, I asked Stephen, "So how do you explain this to people who don't understand it, who may think your experience sounds impossible?"

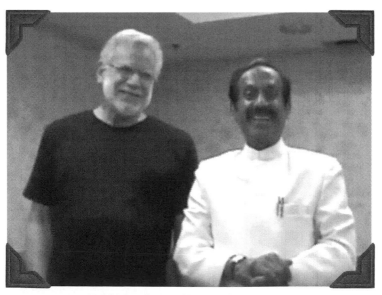

Rabbi Stephen Robbins with Dr. Naram.

"There are multiple means of finding truth," he replied. "There is no such thing as 'bad medicine,' but there is the wrong medicine used at the wrong time and applied in a wrong way. Dr. Naram provides healing support in a way that helps the body, mind, and spirit to heal deeper. Many of Dr. Naram's formulas are 'anti-aging' formulas, although I hate to use that term. It is more about youth-sustaining. In my experience, the healing herbs help the body to produce and burn energy in a healthy rather than self-destructive way. The vigor and the energy I feel as the result of taking them is amazing."

He concluded with these poignant words: "The wisdom of Siddha-Veda is profound, and not just because it is ancient. Simply because something is old doesn't mean it's true or wise. I know some old people who are very foolish, and there are certain old religious beliefs that are very destructive. But there is wisdom, a profound wisdom, in Siddha-Veda that understands the complete makeup of the human being; not from what we now describe in scientific Western terms, but which is understood according to the ancient science. The principles are truly effective for deeper healing, and they are the result of millennia of experience and practice."

> *"The wisdom of Siddha-Veda is profound, understanding the complete makeup of the human being; not from what we could describe in scientific Western terms, but which is understood according to the ancient science."*
>
> –Rabbi Robbins

My Journal Notes

Four Ancient Healing Secrets for Supporting Healthy Hormone Levels in Men (e.g. HGH or Testosterone)*

1) Herbal Remedies—Stephen took some herbal tablets created to support healthy function of hormones, which included ingredients like sesame seeds, tribulus, Indian tinospora, ashwaganda roots, indian kudzu rhizome, and velvet bean seeds.*

2) Marmaa Shakti—On the left forearm, four fingers down from the wrist on the pinky side, press that point 6 times, many times a day.

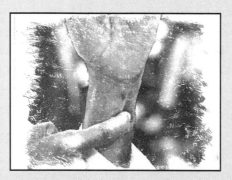

3) Home Remedy—Dr. Naram's Maharaja Secret Home Remedy: Mix and take first thing in the morning 3 almonds (soaked overnight, slide of and discard skins), 3 dates, 3 cardamom pods (soaked overnight, then release inner seeds), 3 tsp. fennel, 1/4 tsp. Brahmi powder, 1/4 tsp. Ashwaganda powder, 1/2 tsp. Kaucha powder, 1/2 tsp. Shatavri powder, & 1 tsp. Cow's Ghee.

4) Diet—Dr. Naram recommends you avoid sour and fermented foods.

*Information (including key ingredients) for herbal formulas mentioned in this book are in the appendix. Bonus Material: To discover more secrets on men's health and virility, please visit the free MyAncientSecrets.com membership site.

Not Everyone Was Happy

After thanking Rabbi Robbins, I went back to the waiting room to see if it was closer to my dad's turn, and there was a swirl of commotion. A man was shouting, "I don't want to wait!" The tension in the room rose with his voice. "Do you know who I am?" he asked. "I am one of the first Indians recognized by Forbes; I've given millions to UCLA's medical school. I don't want to wait."

The other people waiting didn't want to let him go first just because he was rich and noisy, but in order to avoid further distress the attendants snuck him in to see Dr. Naram as soon as possible. Dr. Naram later told me what happened.

From touching his pulse, Dr. Naram told the man about his health problems, the most frustrating of which was a frozen shoulder causing intense pain. The man had tried every other kind of treatment and remedy, with no results. No matter how much he contributed to the prestigious medical school, the doctors could not help him. He was beginning to lose hope that he would ever regain full motion of his arm.

Dr. Naram assured him there was a remedy and proceeded to ask him point-blank, "The question is, what price are you willing to pay?"

The man wasn't surprised. With his good arm he pulled out his checkbook and signed a blank check. "I have already spent so much money on the best medical care with no results. If you fix this, you can name your price. How much do you want? Ten thousand, twenty thousand, fifty thousand?"

Dr. Naram smiled and calmly said, "For everything, there is a price; sometimes we pay with money, sometimes we pay in terms of time or efforts. For this, you cannot pay the price with money. My question for you is, what price are you willing to pay?"

The man looked confused. "I already told you, if you fix it, I will pay you anything. Whatever it takes. I'll pay whatever the price!"

Dr. Naram looked straight at him and said, "Good. If you will do whatever it takes, then . . . will you wait?"

"What do you mean?"

"That is the price you have to pay today," Dr. Naram explained. "You said you would do anything, pay any price; now I am asking you, will you wait?"

"What price are you willing to pay?"
–Dr. Naram

Hesitantly, he agreed, but still wanted more explanation. Dr. Naram said, "Today I want you to wait for . . ." He paused to think, then said, "six hours."

"Can I go to my room to sleep, and then come back?" he asked.

"Sure, go wait for six hours, then come back, and only then we will see if I can help you."

The man emerged from Dr. Naram's office much calmer but confused.

A few moments later my dad's name was called; they said it was almost his turn, so I quickly went to get him.

A Long Six Minutes

My dad tenderly walked with me from the hotel room down the hall to the conference area and to Dr. Naram's door. As we waited outside, he admitted he didn't know how to begin to explain to Dr. Naram everything he was experiencing. All day, he watched people go into and out of Dr. Naram's office, spending only five or six minutes inside. Dad showed me the sheet of paper with the list of his medications and said, "I can't even read this entire list in that short of time."

I had sent a message to Dr. Naram that I was bringing my dad, but said nothing about his condition. I suppose I was testing him. Though I'd already heard and seen many amazing cases, there was still a part of me that wondered, *Was this a hoax?*

I watched my dad walk slowly into the room, slightly hunched over and visibly in pain. Dr. Naram welcomed him with a big smile while I waited anxiously outside.

Though it seemed like forever, only about six minutes later the door opened, and I was surprised by what I saw. My dad looked and walked differently. He held his head higher and stood more upright, with a look of wonder in his eyes.

"How did he know?" my father asked. "That was remarkable, really."

"What happened? What did he know?" I asked.

"I didn't need to say anything to him. Dr. Naram put his fingers on my wrist and, in minutes, described my situation more succinctly and accurately than I ever could. Even if I had my four doctors in the same room to talk about my case, which never happens, they couldn't have described what I'm experiencing as accurately as Dr. Naram just did."

I listened, not knowing what to say or how to process what I felt.

My dad said, "He asked about my profession, too. He seemed genuinely interested and told me it was important work I must do and had to live for. The whole thing was very encouraging! I don't know what to make of it yet, but now I guess we'll see, huh?" He looked around and asked, "What do I do next?"

I was astonished to see the positive impact that being so fully understood had on my dad. He was in a better mood and even started believing that he could be healed. Seeing him in this state of anticipation made my breathing stop. I tried to hide it, but in a matter of moments I went from nervous to elated, and back to nervous again.

Ironically, just as my dad started to feel hopeful, I became hesitant. *Was I misleading my dad and giving him false hope? Did Dr. Naram really have a solution for him? Was I doing the best thing for my dad, or was I wasting the last days of his life chasing a non-existent cure?*

Your Journal Notes

To deepen and magnify the benefits you will experience from reading this book, take a few minutes now and answer the following questions for yourself:

What price are you willing to pay for what you want (in terms of time, energy, efforts, money, discipline, etc.)?

_____

_____

_____

_____

_____

Why is it worth it to you to pay that price?

_____

_____

_____

_____

_____

What other insights, questions, or realizations came to you as you read this chapter?

_____

_____

_____

_____

CHAPTER 8

The Fountain of Youth

There is a fountain of youth: it is your mind, your talents,
the creativity you bring to your life and the lives of the
people you love. When you learn to tap this source,
you will truly have defeated age.

–Sophia Loren

Los Angeles, California

After my father went up to the hotel room to rest, one of Dr. Naram's staff came to me and said, "Dr. Naram would like to speak with you. Do you have a couple of minutes?"

Dr. Naram greeted me with a big smile. "Well, how are you?" he asked, with a bowl of moong bean soup in front of him.

I thanked him for understanding my dad so well and for the hope it gave him. I also wanted to express my concerns, but Dr. Naram interjected, before I managed to get them out, "Your father is amazing, huh? He is a very good man, which helps me understand where you got it from. He has an important mission with children, and I think we can help him. He has work in this life he still needs to complete."

I asked him directly, "Do you think that there is hope for him? Tell me the truth."

"The truth, as I see it, is that your dad has two options. He can continue doing what he is doing and live for a few more months in pain before he passes away. Or he can change his course by using Siddha-Veda's six keys of deeper healing. Doing so, he could live many more years with flexibility, energy, and presence of mind. Which do you prefer?"

"Of course the second option. But how?" I asked, surprised by the confidence Dr. Naram had about my dad's prognosis.

"Do you remember how I met my master?" Dr. Naram asked.

"Yes, how could I forget?"

"How many days did my master tell me to come tomorrow?"

"A hundred days."

"Yes, a hundred days, or three months. For those three months that I was outside his room, I was not just sitting there. I was doing research, like you are doing now. I talked to patients about their problems. I saw people suffering from chronic diabetes, arthritis, heart problems, kidney problems, osteoporosis, different kinds of cancer, liver problems, and many other things. I spoke to people who came back after months or years of doing what Baba Ramdas told them to do, and saw big transformations in them as a direct result of deeper healing. Do you remember how old my master was?"

Before I could answer, he said, "One hundred fifteen years! I was extremely curious by what he was doing differently from others, so I spent the last thirty-six years learning my master's secrets and using them to help people. Would you like to know what, according to him, the secret to the fountain of youth is?"

I nodded. Who wouldn't want to know?

Slowly, he continued, "I'm not exactly sure why I'm sharing this with you, Clint, but I get a feeling perhaps you'll be an instrument in helping many others."

I didn't know how to respond to that. As I was on the fringe of believing him and everything he was saying, a flicker of worry came into my mind that perhaps I'd end up discovering he was a fraud and preying on the hopes of the desperate. The closer I got to him, and the more I started to care, in some ways I also became more guarded. If he was a fraud, would I end up debunking his "clinic" once and for all? Instead of helping him promote his ancient healing method, would I become instrumental in protecting other people from him?

The Ancient Secret for Staying Young

Dr. Naram's face reflected a deep inner peace and confidence as he looked directly into my eyes. He told me that with these secrets, anyone can experience vibrant health, unlimited energy, and peace of mind at any age. He said, "First, you must have a clear idea of what 'youth' is. Only then can you know the secret of staying young."

As Dr. Naram continued, he took out pictures to show me.

"Here is a picture of dear Babaji, one of my master's brothers. He is living in the Himalayas—and is 139 years young."

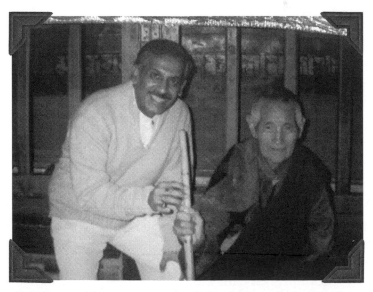

Dr. Naram with a 139-year-young Beloved Master in the Himalayas.

He pulled out another photo. "Here is Sadanand Gogoi, who became Mr. India at sixty-five years young! This is his body now, at the age of seventy."

I stared at the muscular body that looked like it belonged to someone in his forties.

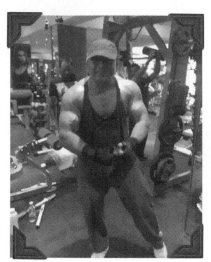 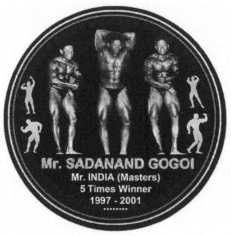

Sadanand Gogoi at 75, Mr. India five-time winner.

Dr. Naram said, "He is using the ancient secrets for building body, muscles, and mind, without damaging his kidneys. The dream of this man, after winning Mr. India, is to compete for Mr. Universe!"

Fondly looking at another picture, Dr. Naram told me about Kusum Atit, who was now eighty-six years 'young.' She was one of his first patients. When she came to him at the age of fifty-six, she could not walk, had high blood pressure, osteoporosis, and arthritis, and was planning on a hip replacement. "What do you think happened to her when she started using the youth secrets?"

I shrugged.

"The woman who could not even walk before won the first prize in a Bombay dancing competition!" he said triumphantly. "I was shocked. I felt joy like you can't imagine!"

He showed me another picture of his master. "This was when he was 115 years young, and I was blessed to have ten years with him

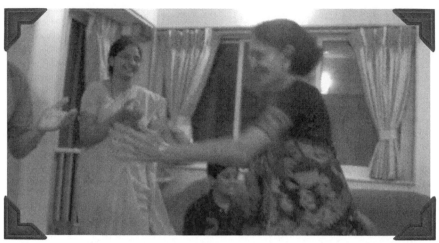

Kusum, 86, dancing with joy after healing her arthritis.

before he left his body. He died at the age of 125. Throughout my training, I received such secrets, wisdoms, powerful insights, and truths from him. Now let me share them with you."

He asked me, "What does 'youth' mean to you, Clint? How do you know if a person is young or old?"

I offered some ideas: "Maybe how they look? Their state of mind? The quality of their skin or their hair?"

Dr. Naram smiled "My master said a person can be twenty years old, or one hundred years young. How can a person be old at twenty, and another, young at one hundred?"

"How?"

"It all depends upon *flexibility*," he said. "Someone can be only twenty years old if he is physically rigid,

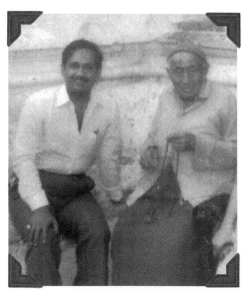

Dr. Naram with his beloved master and teacher, Baba Ramdas.

> *"Youth is a condition achievable at any age when someone is physically flexible, mentally alert and willing to learn, and emotionally full of love."*
>
> –Baba Ramdas
> (Dr. Naram's Master)

mentally stubborn, and emotionally dry. Or, a person can be one hundred years young if he is physically flexible, mentally alert and willing to learn, and emotionally full of love. Interesting, don't you think?"

I paused to take it in. "So 'youth' is about flexibility—in mind, body, and emotions?"

He said, "Yes, Clint, exactly! That's how my lineage understands youth."

I needed clarification. "So the secret to being young at any age is learning how to be flexible?"

He nodded and added that youth is possible at any age if your lifestyle is aligned with your inner nature. "'Young' people are full of hope. 'Old' people lose hope. If you watch the news, everything is about fear, disasters, about a 'hard time that is coming.' So many people project horrible things coming in the future and that makes them anxious. Their life experiences often leave them hurt, afraid, heartbroken, and closed down. To be young at any age is to stay full of hope for the future, hope for yourself, hope for humanity. And you can be 'young' like this, even at 115."

Dr. Naram then said, "Now, the ultimate purpose of the ancient healing secrets my master taught me is this: First, it is about helping people maintain or improve health and flexibility in their body, mind, emotions, and spirit. The ancient tools provide an opportunity to experience deeper healing, and a youthful feeling at any age. Second, this transformation gives people the energy to discover what they want most in their lives. They learn how to align themselves with their inner nature and life's purpose."

"So, if that's your definition of youth," I asked, "I'm still not clear how someone can live to such an advanced age."

"Most anyone can live more than one hundred years if they want to. All you need are Siddha-Veda's six keys of deeper healing."

"What are those six keys?" I asked.

He said, "You've already seen some of the keys at work. Let's see how many you can identify."

"I think one must be home remedies. Like onion rings alleviating my headache. The secret is that anything can be a medicine or a poison if you know how to use it."

"Yes, very good, Clint! And do you remember the secret home remedy for unlimited energy at any age that I gave you during our interview?"

"I don't." Dr. Naram gave me again the 'Super energy drink' home remedy his master was using to feel young at the age of 115 years. This time I took it more seriously.

My Journal Notes

Dr. Naram's Secret Recipe for Super Energy*

Home Remedy—

1) Soak these ingredients overnight in water:

> Raw Almonds 3
> Cardamom 3 pods (or about 30 seeds)
> Fennel seeds 3 tsp.

2) In the morning add:

> 3 Dates (and if you like, 3 apricots, 3 figs),
> 1/4 tsp. cinnamon
> 1/4 tsp. Brahmi powder
> 1/4 tsp. Ashwaganda powder
> 1 tsp. Cow's Ghee
> 2 threads of Saffron

3) Peel off and discard almond skins and cardamon shells (releasing the seeds).

4) Blend or grind all ingredients together with hot water and enjoy.

*Bonus Material: To watch this being made, please refer to the videos in the free MyAncientSecrets.com membership site.

"Is the second instrument related to the herbal formulas?"

"Yes," he replied. "My master taught me secrets about how to grow, harvest, prepare, and combine herbs according to ancient processes that facilitate deeper healing. This is how they become healing herbs."

When he talked about healing herbs, I thought of the tablets gathering dust in a drawer at home, which I had tucked away after only two days of using them. I made a mental note to learn more about them.

"Marmaa is the third instrument of Siddha-Veda," he said. I wrote it down, although I still wasn't exactly sure what it was or how it worked.

"What are the other three?" I asked.

"I will share those with you later. I need to see the rest of the people still waiting. Why don't you come tonight, when I'm finished with the pulse appointments, and witness a marmaa session for yourself?"

I agreed to return, then took my father to the airport.

As we stood at the door of the airport, I gave my dad a hug. We both felt cautiously hopeful about the future. He was determined to do everything Dr. Naram suggested—the diet, the herbs, everything. There was one recommendation, however, that most intimidated him. Dr. Naram invited him to come to India for some in-depth treatments called *panchakarma*.

Before walking in, my dad asked, "Do you want to know the real reason I came with you to LA?"

I shrugged. "It wasn't to see Dr. Naram?"

"No," he shook his head. "I didn't think he would be able to help me. I came because I was worried about what you were getting yourself into."

He hugged me tightly, then looked deep into my eyes and said, "Let's see from here . . . but whatever happens, I hope you know how much I love you."

Your Journal Notes

To deepen and magnify the benefits you will experience from reading this book, take a few minutes now and answer the following questions for yourself:

What does "youth" mean to you? What does it mean to feel young at any age?

_____

_____

_____

_____

_____

If "youth" is about "flexibility," what are some areas in your life you could be more flexible?

_____

_____

_____

_____

_____

What other insights, questions, or realizations came to you as you read this chapter?

_____

_____

_____

_____

_____

CHAPTER 9

Modern Medical Miracles from an Ancient Science?

There are only two ways to live your life. One is as though nothing is a miracle. The other is as though everything is a miracle.

–Albert Einstein

After dropping my dad off, I returned to the hotel for Dr. Naram's marmaa session. I was happy to see that Dr. Giovanni was there too. Even though it was after midnight, Dr. Naram entered the room with a refreshing vitality. Had I not been there all day, I would have never guessed he'd seen over a hundred people that day. He looked as if he was just getting started.

After greeting several people, he walked to the center of the room and asked, "For how many of you is this your first experience with marmaa?"

Almost everyone raised their hands.

"OK, so what is marmaa? It's an ancient technology of deeper transformation, working on all levels of body, mind, emotions, and spirit."

"This ancient technology has nothing to do with religion. Like electricity, it just works, no matter your religion or belief. It is universal."

–Dr. Naram

Dr. Naram said we could read more about this approach to healing in the Mahabharata, one of the major epic Sanskrit texts of ancient India. According to the record, there was a big war that was nothing like modern conflicts. This war had rules. It started and ended at a certain time of day. While the dharma, or duty, of the soldier was to fight, the dharma of healers of Dr. Naram's lineage was to heal. They were not concerned with whether the soldier was a good soldier or a bad soldier—they would help people, no matter who they were, regardless of what side they fought on.

"The healers of my lineage had no enemies, just like we have no religion. Our 'religion' is simply helping humanity."

He described how these masters would go to the battlefield each day after the fighting was over and see who couldn't walk, who'd been hit by arrows, or who had fallen off an elephant and broken a bone. Often, they helped by using marmaa, a technology thousands of years old, to bring instant relief.

"Today, there is no Mahabharata fight, but my job is to make you fit so you can go fulfill whatever your duty in life is."

Dr. Naram explained that in order to understand this ancient technology, which was so powerful, we needed to know that it had nothing to do with religion. "Think of it like electricity," he said. "You turn on the lights and they just work, no matter your religion or belief. The lights don't care if you are Muslim, Christian, Hindu, or atheist. The keys of my healing lineage are also universal. The healing instrument of marmaa can help anyone with chronic and acute challenges, like back pain, stiffness, neck pain, frozen shoulder, pinched nerves, sciatica, ankle pain, knee pain, or even the inability to walk.

"Believe it or not," he said, "in a couple of minutes, marmaa touches the subtle energy points and begins to release the block.

You start to see results and feel less or no pain. How many of you have pain?"

Most people in the room raised their hands.

"I will teach you some marmaas that you can do at home. Some marmaas can be done for you only by me or someone I've trained. What may look like magic at first sight, is a science. The way to benefit from this thousands of years old process is to be clear on what you want. What do you want—from your body, from your mind, from your emotions, from your life? But what if you don't know what you want?" He paused, as some in the audience shook their heads.

"You take most advantage of ancient healing methods by first becoming clear on 'what do you want'?"

–Dr. Naram

"Well, if you don't know, here is the marmaa to discover what you want. Close your eyes. Imagine a white frame over your right eye. Then press on the tip of your right index finger six times. Then ask yourself, 'What do I want?' and see what picture appears in your white frame."

I took a video as Dr. Naram demonstrated the procedure. I was skeptical, not believing that pressing a point on my finger would give me clarity on anything. But when I thought no one was looking, I pressed the point on my own finger just in case it did help. I wasn't aware of anything happening to me other than I was squeezing my finger.

"Most of you are doing it incorrectly. Whenever you do marmaas, sit in the power position—both feet firmly on the ground and back straight."

I was sitting hunched over with my legs crossed, so I sat up straight and put my feet on the ground. Dr. Naram waited until everyone was in this position, then continued, "Now here is a very important point. The 'want' in you has to be a positive anchor. It cannot be what you don't want, or what you are avoiding. Let me give you a very powerful example."

Dreams into Reality

"My mother couldn't walk. She had arthritis, osteoporosis, and degeneration of joints," Dr. Naram said. "Since she couldn't walk, she'd have to use the toilet, bathroom while in bed. That was thirty years ago. I was willing to be a good Indian boy, stay home to clean and feed her every day. But she didn't want our lives to be spent that way."

"I decided to use the ancient methods for her," Dr. Naram continued. "I decided if I could not even help my own mother with them, what good were they?"

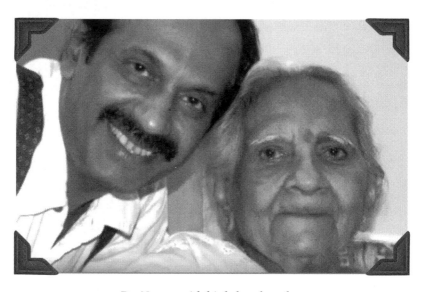

Dr. Naram with his beloved mother.

"Let me share with you a powerful secret my master taught me. The quality of your life depends on the quality of your questions. Most of us ask the wrong questions. I used to ask, 'Why am I fat?' My master said, 'Horrible question, Dr. Naram.' I was focused on what I didn't like. He told me that powerful questions focus on what you want, not what you don't want. So I pressed the point on my mother's finger and asked, 'Mommy, what do you want?'

"The quality of your life depends on the quality of your questions."

–Dr. Naram

"She responded, 'I don't want pain.' Having a 'want' that is negatively framed doesn't work well."

While motioning to his head Dr. Naram said, "There is something known as conscious mind," and motioning near his heart, "then there is subconscious mind." Then, indicating somewhere above his head, "And there is superconscious mind."

"It is this superconscious mind that can guide you if you know how to access it. When you open a clear channel, you are given an answer to the question. Marmaa is a technology to stimulate and make all the powers of consciousness work for you. And one secret is to focus on a positive picture of what you do want, instead of a negative one of what you don't want."

When Dr. Naram pressed the marmaa point again on his mother's finger and reframed the question: "Mommy, if you knew there was no pain, what would you do?"

She said, "I would walk."

Dr. Naram explained that you have to create the future and let go of the past. That is one of the important principles—creating, seeing the future, leaving the past behind, and, at the same time, not losing sight of the present. The reality of Dr. Naram's mother in that moment was that she couldn't walk. She had arthritis and osteoporosis, and even specialists said she couldn't walk. Dr. Naram said again, "But the most important thing was, what did she want?"

Dr. Naram told us that once his mother had an idea of something positive she could envision, he asked her to close her eyes. He pressed another marmaa point farther down on her finger and asked, "If you knew you could walk again, where would you like to go?"

She replied, "I would like to go to the Himalayas."

Each time she gave a response, Dr. Naram would say, "Very good," and pat a marmaa point near her heart six times. He had

"Focus on what you do want, not what you don't want."

–Dr. Naram

her imagine a white frame over her right eye and asked, "Can you see yourself walking in the Himalayas?"

She nodded yes, and he replied, "Very good," patting her heart again.

At that point, Dr. Naram's father, who was watching, got very angry. "'What nonsense! Are you crazy? Why are you giving false hopes to your mother? Your mother cannot walk. You know that. Why are you talking about Himalayas? Forget the Himalayas. She can't even walk to the toilet. She needs knee and hip replacement surgery and you are talking nonsense about the Himalayas. She cannot walk! Why can't you understand this?' he yelled.

Dr. Naram continued, "I said to my father, 'What is important is what your wife, my mother, wants. Not what you think she wants!' My father was a very harsh man and this was the first time I stood up to him.

"My father replied, 'She is an idiot; she does not know what she wants. She doesn't know that she cannot walk.'"

That was too much for Dr. Naram. He looked squarely at his father and said with a firmness that would have made a tiger stop in its tracks, "Get out. She is choosing this. It is her life and her choice."

With that, his father threw his hands up in the air and left the room.

Dr. Naram said, "My father was so angry with me, believing I was cheating my mother by giving her false hope."

Although I didn't speak it out loud, I understood the doubts of Dr. Naram's father. I wondered whether the new hope my dad had would materialize into positive results or was just one more thing he'd be disappointed by.

Dr. Naram described creating a plan for his mom. He consulted his master on which deeper healing secrets could help her walk again. His master told him, "There are two things to consider: one is today and the second is the future. It is important to look at what is happening today but to not let that stop you from believing or seeing how things can be much different and better in the future. Do not get stuck in the reality you perceive today. The journey of a thousand miles begins with a single step. So take that first step, then another, and so on. And soon you may be surprised by where you end up."

During the course of several years, Dr. Naram's mother took certain herbs, changed her diet, and pressed marmaa points regularly while visualizing her dream.

My Journal Notes

Dr. Naram's Secret Recipe for Healthy, Flexible Joints*

1) Home Remedy—Mix the following ingredients and take first thing in the morning: Fenugreek powder ½ tsp., Turmeric powder ½ tsp., Cinnamon powder ¼ tsp., Ginger powder ½ tsp., Ghee 1 tsp.

2) Marmaa Shakti—On the palm of your left hand, between the middle finger and ring finger, count 4 fingers down, and press this point 6 times, many times a day.

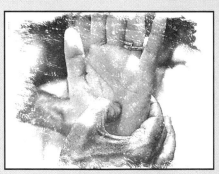

3) Herbal Remedies—Dr. Naram's mother used a cream and took some tablets to support healthy joints, which included ingredients like winged treebine bark, Indian frankincense, chastetree leaves, ginger, and guggul gum resin.*

*Bonus Material: To discover more about ancient secrets for joints, please refer to the free MyAncientSecrets.com membership site.

Then one day, after years of their working together with discipline on her deeper healing plan, Dr. Naram got a phone call from her. "Pankaj, I did it! I'm here in the Himalayas, I'm really here."

She made it to the temple she wanted to visit and camped on one of the peaks. "Although bedridden when she was sixty-seven, now at eighty-two years old, she was hiking the Himalayas," Dr. Naram said. "While others rode horses or were carried on 'balkies' by strong men, she walked. Carrying one small bottle of water in her hand, she was passed by others much younger on horses, who asked, 'What kind of a cheap son do you have that gives you no money for a horse to ride, poor old woman? If your son won't get you a horse, we can pay for you.'"

She said, "No, my son can buy me a horse, but I choose to walk. He is a great son because he gave me the gift of walking."

"That was one of the happiest days of my life." Beaming with moist eyes and a big smile, Dr. Naram said, "She told me, 'I bless you, Pankaj. Share these ancient secrets with everyone, so that you may help others like me.'" Everyone in the room applauded. "The blessing from my mother meant everything to me."

While he was telling the story, I thought about my father's condition and what might be possible for him. I also thought about my mother. I loved her, but I did not understand her. This created conflict sometimes. Listening to Dr. Naram's story I wondered:

> *What did my mom want most in her life? What dream would she like to become reality?*
> *And what would my dad want most if he ever got better? What was his dream?*

Dr. Naram smiled big and said, "My master taught me a priceless secret—that all women are intelligent, and all men are idiots, including me." He laughed. "Do you know what *shakti* is? Shakti is a divine feminine creative power. My master taught me ancient secrets for how any woman can develop the shakti within her. For a man, the moment you respect women, only then you are intelligent, and the shakti also comes to you. Which brings us back to what do *you* want."

Dr. Naram returned to the center of the room and walked everyone through the same steps he'd gone through with his mother, so they could get a clear vision of what they wanted.

"But how does this work?" someone asked. I was wondering the same thing.

Dr. Naram smiled and replied, "Good question. Now, knowingly or unknowingly, we are all programmed. Our subconscious has been programmed by our parents: how to think, how to talk, what to do. We are also programmed by school, by our society, by newspapers, and now by internets. The question is, can we reprogram ourselves to have good health, good vitality, good relationships, good financial freedom? The answer is yes. Marmaa is a technology that helps us reprogram ourselves, to align our lives with our truest purpose. Not only can the pain go away, but you can achieve whatever it is that you want to achieve."

Is that really true?

Have I been programmed by my past to believe or act in certain ways?

If so, is that programming out of alignment with my life's purpose?

Dr. Naram said, "When you discover what you want, it transfers from the conscious mind to the subconscious mind and then to the superconscious mind. Then, creation happens. It is powerful beyond anything you can imagine. I have done it now over a million times. This is my job, my work, my mission, my passion. I only know a few things, and I do them very well. Marmaa is one. And one of the powerful uses of marmaa is to help you discover what you want."

My Journal Notes

Dr. Naram's Marmaa Shakti Secrets for
Discovering What You Want*

1) Close your eyes and imagine a white frame in front of your right eye.

2) On your right-hand pointer finger, press the top portion 6 times, and ask yourself, "What do I want?"

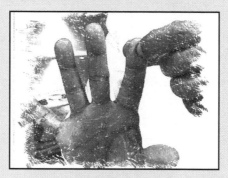

3) Allow any thoughts, feelings, or images to come to you. Write down whatever these are. Tap the left side of your chest with your open right-hand palm 6 times and say, "Very good."

4) On your right-hand pointer finger, press the second (or middle) part of your finger 6 times, and ask yourself, "When I have that, what will I do?"

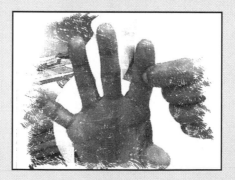

> 5) Allow any thoughts, feelings, or images to come to you. Write down whatever these are.
>
> 6) Tap the left side of your chest with your open right-hand palm 6 times and say, "Very good."
>
> *Bonus Material: To see a video demonstrating this process, please refer to the free MyAncientSecrets.com membership site. (More on this process is found in Chapter 14.)

Then he paused, as if to add something important. "I can help remove the blocks, but you have to see the vision of what you want, what result you want to see in your life, your future. This work must be done by you. In a way, I am like a midwife. I help you deliver, but the baby is born by you. Now, who would like to go first?"

You Can't Get Your Old Wife Back

Lots of hands went up, and Dr. Naram picked Teresa, a woman from Canada in a wheelchair. I had met her and her husband, Vern, earlier that day, and they struck me as the most unlikely couple. Teresa was extremely sweet and intelligent. Vern looked like he should be on the cover of a hunting or fishing magazine, not waiting in an alternative healing setting.

They were both somewhat overweight and I wondered how her disability affected their relationship. From my perspective, it looked like they had a deep connection, the kind most people dream about. Although Vern spent their whole marriage taking care of her, he told me that she was the one taking care of him. Their communication was full of love and respect, and they couldn't keep their hands off each other. They were adorable.

It was Vern's deep love for Teresa that inspired him to search and do anything to help her. They had tried many things he hoped would help her, but to no avail. His love compelled him to bring his wife to LA all the way from Canada, on the chance these ancient methods might help. Earlier in the day I had heard Vern pleading with Dr. Naram many times, "Please, please do something to help my wife." They waited in anticipation for nearly eight hours at the clinic. Now, I watched Vern help Teresa as she struggled to get up out of the wheelchair. He supported her as she hobbled with one crutch in each hand to the center of the room. Her feet were clubbed inward and she couldn't bend her knees, so her walking was more of a waddle. She shifted her weight to one side of her body, then pivoted her hips to swing her other leg forward.

Dr. Naram took her through the same process he had done with his mother, asking Teresa what she wanted. She was clear that she wanted to walk without crutches. Once she could envision it in her mind, Dr. Naram had her lie down on a sheet on the floor. She couldn't get down by herself and was worried she wouldn't be able to get back up. Dr. Naram assured her it was OK, and Vern came to help. As Teresa lay on her back, Dr. Naram motioned to Vern to watch closely. He took a measuring tape and put one end to her navel, then measured the distance to her right toe. "How much is that?" Dr. Naram asked Vern.

"It looks like thirty-six and a half inches."

Then Dr. Naram moved the measuring tape to the end of her left toe. "How much is that?

"That's thirty-nine and a half inches."

"So a three-inch difference! I forgot to tell you," he said to everyone in the room, "an important side effect of coming here is that after marmaa you will feel hormones released that may make you feel very, very happy. So if you don't want to feel happy, please don't come here."

Everyone smiled, especially Teresa.

"Now turn over." He motioned to her to flip onto her stomach. She struggled, but with determination, she made it.

He pressed his fingers on her back in a pattern that was light and gentle, tapping six times in different places. It looked as if he was playing a piano. He asked Dr. Giovanni to lift the shirt from her lower back and put a dab of cream on her skin designed to help with a process called *dard mukti* (pronounced *dahrd mook-tea*). *Dard* can be translated to mean "pain" and *mukti* means "freedom from." This cream was created according to the ancient principles to help relieve different kinds of muscle or joint discomfort. Dr. Naram rubbed it in a circular motion then told her to turn over.

That's it? I wondered. *How could something so quick and gentle make any difference at all?*

Teresa turned over onto her back, and Dr. Naram remeasured her legs.

"How long is the right one?" asked Dr. Naram.

"Thirty-eight inches," said Vern.

"And the left one?"

"Also thirty-eight inches," said Vern, sounding stunned.

Dr. Naram told her how to walk after marmaa, six steps beginning with her right foot. Teresa got up with some assistance, her crutches still lying on the ground, then we all watched with anticipation. Vern stood near, to catch her if she fell, but Dr. Naram told him to go farther away. He had her close her eyes again and see herself walking. He pressed more points behind each knee, then tapped her on the back and said, "Now, walk to your husband." For the first time in years, she took a step without crutches! Then she took another, slowly but straight. She wobbled but kept moving. When she got to Vern, they embraced. The entire room applauded except Vern, whose mouth and eyes were wide open in shock as he hugged her tenderly.

"How do you feel now?" Dr. Naram asked Teresa.

She replied, "Sixty to 70 percent better."

"Really?" Vern asked. She nodded enthusiastically.

Dr. Naram said, "Very good. Now what if you were to do something you haven't done in a long time? What would that be?"

Teresa responded, "Even just sitting down and getting up has been impossible."

Dr. Naram had her close her eyes and visualize herself sitting down and getting up easily without help from her husband.

"I have removed the physical block, but now you have to remove the belief system block. Can you see yourself sitting down and getting up?"

"Yes."

"Very good. Now do it!"

She sat down, awkwardly, then stumbled a little, trying one way, then another, and it worked. She stood up, all by herself.

Vern said, "That is the first time she has done that in over seven years." Everyone applauded.

Dr. Naram said to Vern, "Now you have a new wife. Every morning you will see her happy, enthusiastic. Don't come back to me complaining that your wife is now too young and energetic! Don't say, 'Give me my old wife back.' That's not possible!"

"Thank you very much," Teresa said, with eyes glistening. She walked, without crutches, to Dr. Naram and gave him a most heartfelt hug. A fresh stream of tears flowed down her cheeks as her husband came to wrap his big arms around both of them, holding her close and kissing her forehead. For a moment I thought he was going to kiss Dr. Naram's forehead, too.

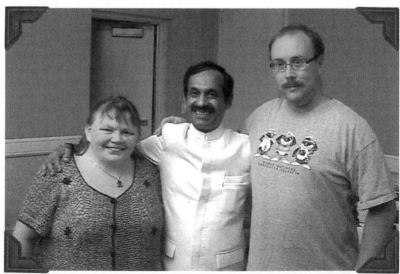

Dr. Naram with Teresa and Vern after her marmaa shakti experience.

Dr. Naram told her, "This feeling or ability will stay. Especially if, in addition to the herbs and diet recommendations, you come for three or four more marmaas in the next months and years. And you can do this one regularly at home." Dr. Naram demonstrated a marmaa everyone could do at home to assist with their deeper healing process.

Dr. Naram asked Teresa to walk again. She did and everyone erupted in applause. We could see the distinct difference from only minutes ago. This was the first time in my life I had seen anything like this, and I didn't know how to take it in. The only stories I heard about crippled or paralyzed people being healed and walking were associated with Jesus. Yet here was Dr. Naram saying that although this looked like a miracle, there was an ancient science behind it. "Sometimes the results are immediate, like with Teresa," he said. "And sometimes they take years of patience and persistence in order to manifest, like the case of my mother. Although the time it takes may differ, the results of deeper healing are predictable."

Then, turning to all of us, he said, "This is real. A real stiffness and block barricaded her ability to walk. Releasing stress, whether it is physical, mental, or emotional, is a phenomenal experience. It is difficult to make sense of such a big change in such a brief moment. If you are in the dark for so long and then there is light, what do you do? It may be disorienting at first, but it is real. Would you like me to share with you what I am doing and how it is working?" Everyone nodded.

Blocks and Breakthroughs

"Let me start with a metaphor. In life, in anybody's life, there are blocks. They can be physical, emotional, relationship, spiritual, financial. When we get blocked, we get stuck, life gets stuck and starts to stink. We can spend five or ten years in that place, making little or no progress. We ask, 'Why are things not happening?' The answer is: we have a block."

Dr. Naram grabbed a chair and put it in the middle of the room. "Let's suppose this chair is a block. If I want to go from here to you, Dr. Clint, I cannot, because there is a block. So, what are the choices? I can go around this way, under, over, or ...?"

"You can remove the block," called out Teresa.

"Exactly. In life, we know there is a block, but most people don't know what type it is. What is the nature of the block? How old is the block? How powerful is the block? Now, with pulse, with marmaa, I am trained to know what that block is."

Dr. Naram continued playfully, "You ask the question, 'Oh, Mr. Block, who are you?'" As he spoke, he pulled out a piece of paper from his pocket. "And suppose this block tells me it is made of paper—simple." He demonstrated tearing the paper with ease and walking through it.

"Easy. But life is not always this simple. Suppose the block tells me it is made of wood. What tools do I need to remove it?"

People shouted out ideas: Saw? Ax? Fire?

"So there are different instruments that can be used. Am I making sense?"

Most people nodded.

"Now suppose the block is made of steel. Do we need different instruments?"

People nodded, yes.

"So in a similar way, there are different marmaas and other instruments to make sure the whole block goes away. You can also think of the block as a door, which just needs you to find the right keys in order to unlock, open, and move beyond it. For example, for joint pain like my mother had, there is the remedy of ghee. If a door creaks, what do we do? We give it oil. So we can ask ghee, 'Oh Mr. Ghee, who are you?' Then the ghee responds: 'I am lubricating and rejuvenating. I am reducing or balancing vata, pitta, and kapha. I make your skin glow without make-up, soothe your emotions, improve your sleep, and help your joints work smoothly.' Ghee is magical. My master once told me that I should never steal anything, yet if I must steal something, it would be ghee. He wasn't telling me to steal, just emphasizing how important cow's ghee is.

My Journal Notes

Magical Benefits of Cow's Ghee*

Among many other benefits, it can help with:

- lubricating and rejuvenating your body, mind, and emotions;
- balancing vata, pitta, and kapha;
- making your skin glow without make-up;
- soothing your emotions;
- improving sleep;
- helping your joints work smoothly;
- plus many, many more . . .

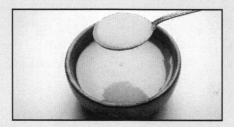

Two Home Remedies Using Ghee to Unlock Its Many Benefits in Your Life:

1) For supporting great joints, skin, digestion, and brain power, take 1 tsp. ghee first thing in morning on an empty stomach, and 1 tsp. at night.

2) For great sleep: take a bit of ghee on your first two fingers and rub in circular clockwise motion on your temples. With your pointer finger, press the temples 6 times.

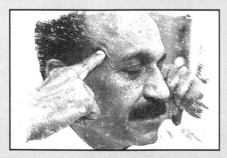

*Bonus Material: To see a recipe for making ghee according to a special ancient process and some interesting scientific studies about how eating moderate amounts of Ghee doesn't appear to increase cholesterol, please visit the free MyAncientSecrets.com membership site.

"No matter the nature of the block, there are six keys of deeper healing to remove it and rebalance your system. Many people try to find a shortcut or a quick fix, searching for the cheapest or fastest solution. Usually, it doesn't work. On the contrary, it can make things worse!"

"What do you mean?" Teresa asked.

"Let me give you a practical example. My father had high blood pressure and diabetes—it runs in my family. What do most people do? They take a medication that suppresses the symptoms instead of removing the block. It does not make you free from diabetes or high blood pressure or whatever the problem is. You still have diabetes or high blood pressure. All you do is suppress the symptoms and often end up with side effects."

Dr. Giovanni then spoke up to add a point: "As an allopathic doctor, I had similar situations with many patients who were taking modern medications."

"What does 'allopathic doctor' mean?" Teresa asked.

"Good question. 'Allopathy' or 'allopathic medicine' is another name for Western modern medicine. I was trained at a modern medical university in Italy as this kind of a doctor, and while giving these kinds of modern medications, I realized I was not helping patients come out of the problem, the block. I was only numbing the pain or suppressing the symptoms. Allopathy is good, but modern medicine is not the final authority. It does a good job with many things, but ultimately your body and your health are your responsibility. Do you ask what the side effects of treatments given to you might be, like what negative things may also come as a result of the drugs or surgery? Do you research to see if you have other options? There is nothing wrong with modern allopathic medicine or any healing path. It is your choice. Just make sure you ask enough questions to know the ramifications of each option, in order to make the right choice for you."

Dr. Naram turned to me, though he spoke to everyone. "My two uncles didn't know they had a choice. They were on heavy medications for high blood pressure and diabetes, until they died young of a stroke, kidney failure, and brain damage. Seeing this, my father, who I had difficulties with my whole life, finally said, 'No, I do not want a shortcut that only suppresses the symptoms. Pankaj, can you help me? I choose to discover a way to become healthy, to reverse diabetes, reverse blood pressure, and become strong.' When the ancient healing methods worked for him, he went back to being frustrated with me, this time saying, 'Why did you not meet your master ten years earlier? Why did you not convince me sooner that this could work? I could have avoided so much suffering and done so much more!'" Dr. Naram laughed at the memory.

"To achieve what my father did, he needed to completely remove the block, and for that you need the right keys. Without drugs and without surgery, my masters have been successfully removing the blocks that cause everything from high blood pressure, diabetes, and autism to cancer and depression."

"What are the six keys of deeper healing?" Teresa asked.

"Very good question. One is marmaa. Another one is home remedies—how to see anything as a medicine or poison, depending on how you use it. And diet—knowing which foods either create blocks or help to remove them. If you want to go faster and deeper, there are certain healing herbal formulas that work according to the ancient science of healing people deeper and deeper. They are not intended to be a quick fix, but long term. They are very safe and work in subtle but profound ways by addressing the root problems. They remove blocks and rebalance your body so it can work naturally in the way it was meant to."

The explanation regarding blocks was simple enough, but I still didn't understand how this ancient science helped resolve so many problems that Western science was apparently just suppressing.

"*Shakti* is our word for 'power,' the divine power to do things or create things. It is already in you. Marmaa goes inside and helps to bring it out. The healer is just a midwife, but you deliver your own baby. Marmaa works with the other keys so you can experience vibrant health. Every day, I thank my master for teaching them to me."

"Shakti is power, already inside you. Marmaa goes inside and helps to bring it out. The healer is just a midwife, but you deliver your own baby."

–Dr. Naram

Dr. Naram continued working on person after person. Finally, there was only one person left— the wealthy man with the frozen shoulder who had been asked to wait six hours.

Removing the Blocks That Cause Pain

When Dr. Naram had first walked into the room, I saw this man get up to meet him. I overheard Dr. Naram quietly ask him again how much he wanted relief from his frozen shoulder, and what price he was willing to pay.

"I told you I am willing to pay any price, only you wouldn't take my money."

Dr. Naram said, "Yes, you can't buy this with money. I'm very proud that you paid a price in terms of time. Now, for deeper healing, you will need to pay the price in terms of service. You will be the last one I will help tonight, and you will first serve everyone here." The man's wife looked shocked, and we all watched with varying degrees of surprise as her husband helped other people all night with their shoes, getting them water, holding the measuring tape, and genuinely finding ways to assist those who came before him. At almost two in the morning, after everyone else had left, it was finally his turn.

Dr. Naram proceeded to do two different marmaas on him. For the first one, he had the man lie on the floor like Teresa. For the second one, he had him sit on a chair, facing backward. Before Dr. Naram started the second marmaa, he asked the man to raise the arm with the frozen shoulder as high as he could. He could bring it up only about halfway before he yelped, "Ouch!"

When asked how long he'd experienced this problem, the man replied that it had been years. Dr. Naram inquired whether he wanted to lift his arm six inches higher. The man nodded, saying he would love that.

Dr. Naram asked him to close his eyes and visualize himself lifting his arm six inches higher. "Can you see yourself, in your mind, lifting your arm six inches higher?" he asked.

He quietly said yes.

Dr. Naram tapped the man's forehead, saying, "Very good." He pressed some points, adjusted the man's neck, and moved his arm back until there was a light click. Dr. Naram asked him to raise his arm, and he began to do so. He got to the point where he stopped before, with a look on his face that anticipated resistance and pain. That look melted away into an expression of pure surprise when his arm continued to lift. He watched with all of us in amazement as his arm went straight above his head, now fully mobile.

The man brought his arm down and tried lifting it again to make sure it was real. Again, full range of motion. "I can't believe it, I can't believe it," he repeated. His wife walked up to give him a hug, astonished by the change. It wasn't just the lack of pain. Her husband's agitation and anger melted into softness, kindness, and gratitude.

I wondered on how many levels of healing Dr. Naram was working, and how this deeper healing went beyond the physical ailment or manifestation.

Each experience that night left me with a deepened sense of possibility and awe. As I witnessed so many varied examples of transformation, my thoughts were shifting. I was less concerned about this being real and more curious about how this ancient healing system worked. Inevitably, I wondered, *Would it work for my dad?*

An Unexpected Invitation

Once the marmaa session was complete, I asked Dr. Naram if I could show him some of the video footage I'd taken during the day. As he watched each person share their experience, Dr. Naram's smile spread even wider than normal.

I saw how emotional he became, hearing their stories. He said tenderly, "Now, maybe, you can begin to understand why I love my work and how I can sleep so well at night."

He looked straight at me and asked, "Clint, do you know what one of the greatest things about you is, one of your greatest strengths?"

I was taken aback. We didn't know each other that well. How could he know my strengths? "What?" I asked.

"You have a presence that opens people up."

Receiving compliments isn't something I do well, so I didn't know how to respond. "Really?" I quietly replied.

"Yes, I've been watching you, and I've been testing you. I have been asking people to speak with you and come back afterward to report to me."

I didn't know what to think. He was testing me? I thought I was testing him. I suddenly felt self-conscious that he was testing me without my knowledge or permission. At the same time I was curious why he was thinking about me enough to want to "test" me in the first place, and what the results of his "testing" showed him.

He continued, "Your being, who you are, allows people to open up and share their lives, their experiences."

There was an awkward silence. I tried to respond, but nothing came out. I never thought of myself in this way before.

Then he looked at me again and said, "Where do you go after this?"

"I go back to my postdoctorate work and research in Finland," I said.

Dr. Naram said, "Good. I go to Europe very soon, too. I'll be visiting Germany, Italy, and France. Would you like to see something truly amazing?"

"What do you have in mind?"

"Can you meet me in Europe?" He pulled out his schedule.

I looked at my own schedule and saw I had some dates free while he was in Italy. Curious as I was, I didn't know how my interest in what he was doing fit into the rest of my life. And the truth was that although I hoped it would help my dad, I still had doubts about it because it contradicted so much of what I'd been taught since I was young.

Dr. Naram noticed my hesitation. "If you do come, it will be one of the most amazing experiences of your life."

Your Journal Notes

To deepen and magnify the benefits you will experience from reading this book, take a few minutes now and answer the following questions for yourself:

What percent of the time do you focus on what you don't want versus what you do want?

_____

_____

_____

Follow the process outlined in this chapter for discovering what you want. After you press the marmaa point and ask the question, what is the first thing that comes into your mind—what do you want?

_____

_____

_____

When you have that, what will you do?

_____

_____

_____

What other insights, questions, or realizations came to you as you read this chapter?

CHAPTER 10

_____

_____

_____

Can a Menopausal Woman After 50 Have a Baby?

*In conflict between the heart and the brain,
follow your heart.*

–Swami Vivekananda (Indian mystic, 1863-1902)

Milan, Italy

I've been blessed. Even though my parents never had a lot of money, I was able to find scholarships, work, and ways to travel. My soul has always been drawn to traveling. When asked why I liked it so much, I'd respond, "I feel alive when I see how people around the world live their lives differently." And that's true. I am driven to understand more about what is human versus what is my culture. Immersing myself in other cultures is the fastest way to discover what I can't immediately see about myself.

What I wouldn't tell people—and didn't consciously understand at the time—was that traveling was also a convenient way to distract myself from fears about my past and future. It diverted me from my own discomforts and self-perceived inadequacies.

Italy was one of my favorite places to run to. And for good reasons: the gelato, the pizza, the artwork, the gelato, the language, the pasta, the gelato, the chocolate, the people . . . Did I mention the gelato?

I flew from Helsinki to Milan and took the bus to the main train station. Stately marble arches, robust statues, intricately passionate paintings, delicious smells, and energetic voices all welcomed me to Italy.

Dr. Giovanni arranged for a car to pick me up. Soon after I arrived, a little red convertible pulled up.

"Ciao!" said the driver, a friendly Italian who introduced himself as Luciano. He had a big mustache curled at the tips, spoke with a thick Italian accent, and was dressed in a yellow sports jacket and suspenders, all topped with a white-brimmed hat. Handing me a daffodil, he said, "Buongiorno! Big welcome from Milano to you!"

The melodious way he spoke sounded as if he'd burst into a song at any moment. I thanked him and soon we were on our way to where I'd be staying for the next few nights. He didn't speak much English, and I spoke even less Italian, but somehow we understood each other.

We drove past ornate churches, bustling cafés, and a quaint park that had a castle-like structure with a brimming fountain in the middle. We arrived at a charming, tranquil house lined with white pillars and green vines winding up and down its walls. Inside this humble, cozy home, delicious fruits, dark chocolates, and hot herbal tea were waiting for me. By the time I went to sleep, all my senses were drenched in beautiful Italy.

Can You Have a Better Sex Life in Your Eighties Than Newlyweds Do?

Early the next morning, I set out for the clinic that was hosting Dr. Naram. I was shown to the room I'd use to interview people, and I set up my video camera and settled in. I realized that what started out in India as recording stories just to create a gift for Dr. Naram had transitioned in LA into an effort to gain more information and evidence that could help my father. In Italy, this was the first time whereby documenting the cases of people, I felt like I was a semi-official part of the team. Even if I was just volunteering, it felt like what I was doing might have more value than I originally thought.

Dr. Naram arrived with incredible vitality and wonder, as if it were the first day of his life and everything was new and colorful. He greeted me, asked about my father, and told me how happy he was I could come.

Dr. Giovanni greeted me with a kiss on both cheeks and a big hug. He held both my arms with his hands so tightly, I had no-where to go. He gazed into my eyes with a warm smile on his face. Normally, I'd feel uncomfortable looking into someone's eyes for so long, but feeling his love and kindness melted my awkwardness and surrendered me into the moment. No words were needed to express his feelings, and it was nice to know he was pleased I could join him in his homeland.

The waiting room began to fill up. As people filtered in, my dreamy state from being in such a beautiful place slowly faded as I witnessed the intensity of the pain many were experiencing.

One elderly woman with disfigured fingers and hands gripped her walker as she painstakingly struggled to enter the room. Another man was breathing heavily and arduously with the assistance of an oxygen tank his son carried with him. A woman with tears in her eyes held her baby in her arms, but I couldn't tell why she was crying. Another young mother came in with two children: one with Down Syndrome and the other with a severe skin problem.

At that time, the economy in Italy was far from rosy. Many businesses closed down and approximately twenty percent of young adults were unemployed. Conventional health care was covered by the government, but insurance plans didn't accommodate ancient healing methods, so people had to pay out of pocket. It cost about seventy euros (approximately $100 USD) for their consultation with Dr. Naram, plus about two to five euros per day (three to seven USD) for the herbs they received afterward. Yet, day after day, crowds eagerly waited to see him.

I was extremely curious why so many Italians were lining up to see Dr. Naram. What inspired them to choose this?

The first person Dr. Naram introduced me to was a young man who first came to him nineteen years prior as a toddler. At that time, his parents were told by doctors that his kidneys were undeveloped and failing, that he needed dialysis and would soon need a transplant. He had polycystic kidney disease, and most people with this condition struggle immensely in life. After many years, with Dr. Naram's help, tests showed his kidneys were normal without needing dialysis or a transplant!

"Last time, he asked me if he could have a girlfriend," said Dr. Naram. "I said, 'Of course, why not?' He said, 'But Dr. Naram, I have a kidney problem.' I said, 'No, you *had* a kidney problem.'" He laughed with joy at the result.

Dr. Giovanni told me, "The health of this boy is remarkable; he is looking very good. And the boy told us proudly that he now has a girlfriend!"

Then an elderly couple in their eighties came, talking with contagious Italian enthusiasm. They couldn't speak much English, but a kind woman at the clinic translated for me. They shocked me by sharing that not only was their age-related joint pain almost gone and their digestion better, but they also experienced something most people half their age only dreamed of. They said they had a better sex life than newlyweds! The elderly woman shared all the details, which I didn't need to know, but that didn't stop her. She told me how she had felt dryness and pain in her vagina. She had no desire to kiss or be held, avoiding her husband, who was also having problems. "Now we can't keep our hands off each other! I love to touch him and love when he touches me!"

She said the diet, herbs, and home remedy Dr. Naram prescribed improved her hormone levels and naturally increased lubrication, so she felt more pleasure in every aspect of her life. She then said

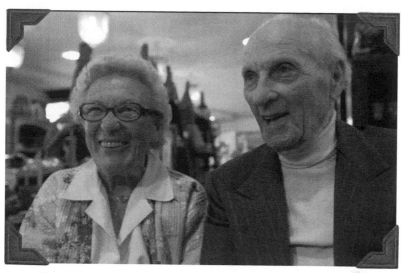

Elderly Italian couple, in love and able to express it in every way.
Photo captured by Fabio Floris and Andrea Pigrucci.

something that made the translator's eyes open wide as she let out a laugh of surprise. After a pause to catch her breath, she translated it. This elderly woman explained with such fervor how they now had sex at least three times a week.

I couldn't help but laugh, too. It was awkward hearing this grandmother talk about sex, but her enthusiasm made it feel innocent and beautiful. She even knew exactly what time of morning her husband was most likely to have an erection so she could be ready for him.

"What good is it if I can only eat pasta, pizza, but not enjoy my husband as a lover? We are more in love than ever and enjoy showing it to each other, with vigor!" I'm sure I was blushing, and hoped my smile would hide it.

Their story intrigued me because I knew male friends in their twenties and thirties who had problems with erectile dysfunction, which impacted their self-confidence. They felt powerless and embarrassed. And here was an eighty-seven-year-old man and an eighty-one-year-old woman having sex multiple times a week!

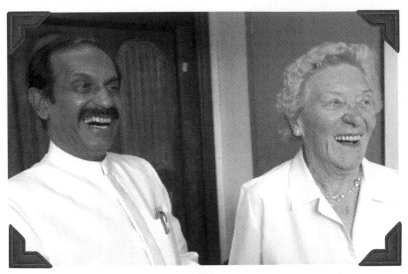

Dr. Naram laughing with surprise and joy as this elderly Italian
woman describes the youthful experience of her new life.
Photo captured by Fabio Floris and Andrea Pigrucci.

Coming Out of Menopause to Have a Baby?

After this interview, Dr. Naram came to tell me I must speak with
a woman named Maria Chiara. Maria was tall, with dark hair and
bright eyes. She told me her story of how she first came to Dr.
Naram three years earlier.

"Dr. Naram asked me, 'What do you want?' I told him I wanted
my periods back so I could have another child. I knew I was asking
the impossible, but wanted it anyway."

"At the time I was already in menopause and hadn't had a period for three years," she said. "When menopause started, I felt depressed and had mood swings. I had pain everywhere and couldn't
sleep. My whole body was on fire from hot flashes. At night, I had
to open windows because I was sweating like crazy. I'd try to sleep,
changing my pillows, sheets, and position, but I couldn't fall asleep.
I was so tired, and experiencing bloating, cramps, and indigestion.
I also had dryness in my vagina, and no libido. The old woman
came out of me, and my skin was crawling. Then the dizzy spells

started—I'd walk and the whole world started to spin. I needed to pee many times a day, and during the night. To remedy that, I had to wear pads. Back pain started, and noise in the bones, which my doctors told me was osteoarthritis. I felt old. And worst of all, I started growing hair in my weird places. But then I got a new boyfriend who is younger than me and, although we have some challenges, I have a big wish to have a child with him."

"Her case reminded me of another woman who came once," Dr. Naram told me. "She said Jesus came in her dream and told her Dr. Naram could help her come out of menopause. Surprised, I told her, 'Jesus may have come in your dream, but he did not come in my dream.'" Dr. Naram laughed. While helping that woman, Dr. Naram discovered secrets that he felt could also help Maria.

When she first came to him, Dr. Naram had told Maria, "You are a very good woman. The problem is not you. Who you are is something different. It is your hormones causing your hot flashes, bloating, anger, and agitation. Your boyfriend may think you are an angry woman, but that is not who you are. He does not understand. You may be feeling guilty and confused, but again, your imbalanced hormones are creating this havoc, not you."

He warned Maria that the secrets could also cause some side effects, like more young men wanting her. "My original master, Jivaka, was treating Amrapali, who at age sixty was considered the most beautiful woman in the world and kept attracting younger men. Even the thirty-five-year-old king, who already had a younger wife, wanted to marry her."

"I can't promise anything regarding having a baby," he told her, "but according to these ancient secrets I can definitely help you look and feel younger. And we can see what else comes with it. Are you willing to take that risk?"

"What happened?" I asked.

She told me she followed the diet diligently and took all the home remedies and herbs for about one year. With a huge smile of total bliss, she said, "Now I am fifty-six years old, and my menstrual cycle has started again!"

Dr. Giovanni couldn't help but smile, too, adding that he was doubtful when Dr. Naram spoke with Maria three years earlier. He had seen younger patients go into menopause and get their cycle back, but never a woman her age. "From a medical standpoint," he said, "this was unprecedented and amazing."

Maria added, "I can create now, I can have a child. I feel like I'm in heaven!"

I asked her, "Do you have any proof of your age, like your driver's license?"

With a big smile, Maria pulled out her purse and showed me her picture and the date of birth on her driver's license, saying, "The herbs helped me look and feel younger. Everyone I meet guesses that I am around forty. Even my boyfriend gets jealous when younger men look at me. I am proud of how I feel now."

Dr. Giovanni added, "I am very proud of her because she had such a strong faith and desire. Even when most people believe that you can't get pregnant once you go into menopause, she believed she could. She chose a different path for herself. She followed the protocol and as a result has achieved a remarkable thing."

Hearing these comments, Dr. Naram said, "My master, wherever he is, must be feeling so good about how the ancient healing secrets he gave me are helping Maria. She is achieving her dreams! Can I share with you another case like this one?"

I nodded.

"There is another woman in Paris who I want you to meet. Hélène came to me when she was nearly fifty. Her periods had stopped for six years and yet when I asked her, 'What do you want?' she said, 'I really want to have a baby.' At this point I said, 'Very good,' only Dr. Giovanni, who was with me at the time, said, 'What do you mean?' and pulled me aside. He said, 'Dr. Naram, you do not understand. She has been in menopause for six years! There is no way she can have a baby. Why would you give her a false hope?' I told him this was not about what he wanted or thought was possible, but about what this wonderful woman wanted. I gave her all the ancient secrets, the home remedies, herbal formulas, diet, everything, and she was disciplined. She followed it exactly, with patience and persistence. Then, believe it or not, I got a call from her. She was so happy and when I asked why, she said she was now getting cramps. Amazing, huh? Being excited about getting cramps. I told her it was a good sign and to continue. Then a few months later, she called me again. She said, 'Dr. Naram, I started having periods again, like when I was twenty years old!' This was a celebratory moment for both of us—I can't put it in words. I wanted to dance and cry. It worked!

"She was excited she could have a baby now but said there was another problem. I asked, 'What problem?' She said, 'Dr. Naram, I don't have a boyfriend!'" Dr. Naram's eyes were wide open as he told this part of the story. "Even this obstacle did not stop her, as she knew emphatically what she wanted. And she found her own way to get pregnant with artificial implantation. The next time I came to Paris, she brought with her a healthy, wonderful baby girl! She said it was a miracle of both ancient and modern science. The joy and satisfaction I felt in seeing her dream come true, of her holding this beautiful baby, was unimaginable! It was better than winning a Nobel Prize."

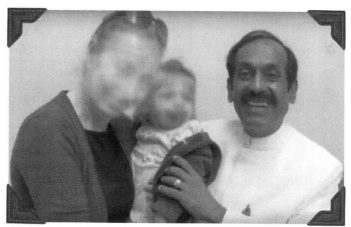

Dr. Naram in Paris with Hélène, 52, and her beautiful baby girl.
She did not want to be recognized so we blurred her image, but she agreed
that this picture contained so much joy it should be in this book.

Dr. Naram expressed gratitude for his master, who taught him this ancient science, and this woman's faith and persistence, which

"Fennel is a woman's best friend. It naturally supports great estrogen and progesterone levels."

–Dr. Naram

produced such amazing results. He was thrilled with the power of the herbal formulas and simple home remedies he gave her, like cumin powder, ajwain powder, hing, dill seed powder, black salt, alum, and fennel. "Fennel is a woman's best friend. It naturally supports great estrogen and progesterone levels."

Dr. Naram emphasized that his master taught him: "When you have a burning desire, with big faith, commitment, and discipline, then anything is possible."

So many questions whirled through my mind about the methods he used to get the results that I had seen working in India, the United States, and Italy. Whereas before it was about 80 or 90 percent, my skepticism was now at about 30 percent. My questions and curiosity were around 65 percent. The remaining 5 percent revealed that cracking through the surface of my thoughts was a confidence and trust in this ancient healing method.

"How did you help these women to have their periods again after menopause?" I asked Dr. Naram. "And what exactly did you do to help that elderly couple to become so youthful again, like newlyweds?"

"When you have a burning desire, with big faith, commitment, and discipline, then anything is possible."

–Baba Ramdas
(Dr. Naram's Master)

"You really want to know?" Dr. Naram asked me.

"Yes!" I said.

"Well, I really want you to know. From my heart to your heart, Clint, I want you to know how this works."

"Then, please, tell me."

"For that, you will need to come tomorrow."*

Bonus Material: In order to discover Amrapali's Secret Remedies and how this elderly couple remained so youthful. Dr. Naram felt that giving you more context and support would be helpful. For that, please see the appendix and the free videos in the MyAncientSecrets.com membership site.

Your Journal Notes

To deepen and magnify the benefits you will experience from reading this book, take a few minutes now and answer the following questions for yourself:

What burning desires do you have in your heart, even if to some they may seem like impossibilities? (If you do not judge yourself or your desires as being right or wrong, good or bad, possible or impossible, and you do not worry about what others think of it, then what do you discover that *You* really want?)

_____

_____

_____

_____

_____

What other insights, questions, or realizations came to you as you read this chapter?

_____

_____

_____

_____

_____

CHAPTER 11

A Secret Diet for Living to Over 125 Years of Age?

The doctor of the future will give no medicine, but will interest his patient in the care of the human frame, in diet and in the cause and prevention of disease.

–Thomas Jefferson (3rd president of the United States of America, & principal author of the Declaration of Independence)

The next day I spoke with Simone Rossi Doria, the man who coordinated logistics on the tour for Dr. Naram. "Italy was the first country outside India where Dr. Naram shared his ancient healing system. That was over twenty-five years ago," he said proudly. Indeed, some ninety-five people visited Dr. Naram the day I was at his clinic in Milan. How did all these Italians know about him? "Word of mouth, email lists, and newspaper articles did a lot to spread the word," Simone told me.

He shared that thousands upon thousands of Italians from more than sixty cities already benefited from Dr. Naram's clinics. Several Italian doctors were trained by Dr. Naram in the ancient methods, and it all started with Simone's sister, Susi.

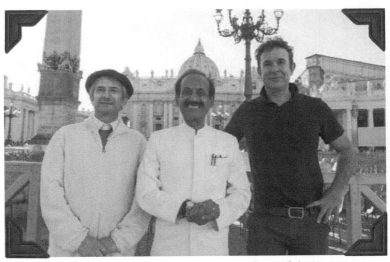

Dr. Giovanni, Dr. Naram, and Simone in front of the Vatican.

I met Susi and their mother during a food break later that day. She was a thoughtful woman who gained a lot of experience thanks to her love of traveling and openness to life. Pucci, their mother, was full of energy, enthusiastic, and vibrantly expressive. Originally from England, Pucci had married an Italian and lived in Italy for so long that she now spoke Italian fluently.

Susi and Dr. Naram's father were staying during the same time at the Sathya Sai Baba ashram in India in 1987. One day, Dr. Naram went there to visit his father. A group of Italians became interested in him and his work and Susi translated for them. When she asked him to check her pulse, he diagnosed a liver problem and told her she had hepatitis A. She didn't believe him and insisted she felt fine. Ten days later, her eyes turned yellow.

Susi's mom said, "Susi thought she had food poisoning, due to some fish she'd eaten before leaving Italy. She went for a blood test, which confirmed she had hepatitis A. She could not believe Dr. Naram knew long before the blood test, just by checking her pulse. How could he have known?"

Susi explained how she understood the method now from hindsight. "Instead of taking a blood test and running an exam, he can read the signals in your pulse. Through the pulse diagnosis, Dr.

Naram is able to understand what is wrong in your body. I know many doctors are skeptical of this, but I have seen many like me who went to Dr. Naram and had the same experience. After meeting him, they took blood tests and did other exams, confirming what he had already diagnosed through only the pulse. It takes many years to master this skill, because it is both an art and a science. Through the fingers, you can know what level the vata, the pitta, the kapha are. You can feel if there is an imbalance, and if you go deeper, you can understand if there is a block and where it is."

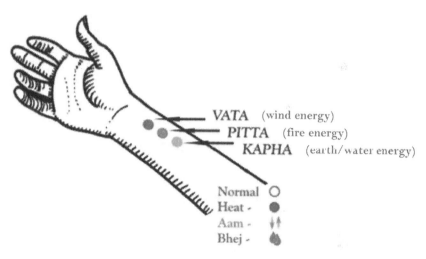

VATA (wind energy)
PITTA (fire energy)
KAPHA (earth/water energy)

Normal O
Heat - ●
Aam - ♦♦
Bhej - ♦

Diagram of some of the basic elements which can be detected when taking a pulse. The strength, pattern, and speed of the pulse in each point indicates any potential imbalances and blocks in the person's system. Those blocks and imbalances correlate to physical, mental, and/or emotional problems that person is facing, or will likely face in their future.

Dr. Giovanni had already explained the concept of doshas to me, and after doing my own research, I knew that Susi was talking about the elemental aspects of the body that both Siddha-Vedic and Ayurvedic approaches to healing are based on. Vata is the wind energy, pitta is fire, and kapha is water/earth. Each person's constitution is different, depending on which quality, or combination of qualities, is predominant. Based on how they manifest in the pulse, imbalances can be detected and illnesses diagnosed.

Susi was supposed to fly home to Italy the next day, but Dr. Naram and his wife, Smita, convinced her to stay in his home, as she was too weak to fly. This provided her an opportunity to change her diet and to take the herbal formulas Dr. Naram created for her.

Although most people can work through many of their challenges without going anywhere, in extreme cases, or when someone is seeking faster progress, they can go for *panchakarma* (pronounced *pahnch-ah-kahr-mah*), or *asthakarma* (pronounced *ahst-ah-kahr-mah*). Both are multiprocess cleansing methods for rebuilding of the body's core systems. *Karma* means "action," and *pancha* means "five." Panchakarma consists of five actions to remove toxins from the body. In asthakarma, there are eight actions, or three additional steps, to cleanse, purify, and rebalance the body from the inside out.

As Susi talked about being in India and receiving such good care from Dr. Naram and his wife, Smita, I thought about my dad. Two weeks earlier I had called him and discovered he had received the delivery of herbal formulas. Just by changing his diet and taking the herbs regularly, he felt a little less pain and more energy, and it gave him hope. He surprised me by saying, "Son, I think I'm starting to wrap my mind around the idea of a flight to India." I immediately booked his flight and his spot at the Ayushakti clinic in Mumbai for the month-long panchakarma treatments Dr. Naram recommended. At about the same time I arrived in Italy, my dad landed in India. The flight was hard for him. He was so weak when he got off the plane in Mumbai, two kind Muslim gentlemen he'd flown with had to hold his arms to make sure he didn't topple over. When I received his email telling me he felt as if he was cared for by angels, and had settled into the clinic, I was grateful. I was also anxious about what his experience would be like going forward.

In Italy, as I listened to Susi, she said that after just a couple of weeks into her treatments, she saw enough improvement with the special diet and herbs Dr. Naram gave her to head home. When she arrived back in Italy, her first blood test showed something remarkable: her liver was healthy.

"My doctors in Italy told me this kind of toxicity from food usually takes several months to recover from," she said. "When they tested me after one month and saw my liver was functioning perfectly, they were shocked. I told them about Dr. Naram's deeper methods, his ancient formulas, the herbal food supplements and diet recommendations, and they wanted to learn more."

To thank him for helping her, Susi asked Dr. Naram to come and do a seminar on his healing methods in Italy. It took him a while to find time, but thanks to her persistent requests, he agreed. Dr. Naram and his wife, Smita, arrived in Italy in 1988 on May 4, his birthday.

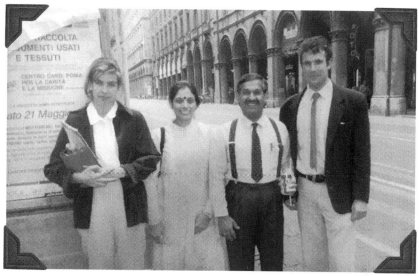

Dr. Naram's first time in Italy, with his wife Smita, Susi and Simone Rossi Doria. (1988)

From India to Italy

Dr. Naram walked in to get some moong soup and saw us there. Susi said, "We are telling Clint about your first visit to Italy."

Dr. Naram laughed and said, "It was my first visit to Europe, and everything seemed strange compared to India. No one spoke English, and as I began speaking at the seminar Susi created, everyone looked at me funny."

With Susi translating, Dr. Naram asked the audience if anyone had ever heard of Siddha-Veda or Ayurveda before. No one raised their hand. He asked if they were interested, and not one hand went up. This made him slightly nervous, so he asked a different question "How many of you are interested in living up to one hundred years?" Only one person raised their hand. Dr. Naram was desperate, but Susi encouraged him to tell his personal healing story, so he did. Dr. Naram spoke about meeting his 115-year-young master and how part of his secret to long life entailed mostly avoiding cheese, tomatoes, wheat products, and alcohol.

The crowd erupted. One man stood up and shouted, "What? No wine, no cheese, no pasta? This is not acceptable!" Someone else added, "Horrible! I eat cheese, pasta, and pizza every day! And I drink wine."

As Dr. Naram recounted the story, he set down his moong soup so he could wave both his hands while speaking with a semi-Italian accent over his Indian accent, which was hilarious. He now understood the Italian culture better and could laugh at the awkwardness of the situation all those years ago.

"I had left India for the first time to share my secrets, and it seemed as if no one was interested. I did not speak the language, but I could tell that whatever I was saying was not working, and my heart was starting to sink." He looked at me and asked: "So now, Clint, what would you do?"

I shook my head.

"I am smiling now, but in that moment, I was not. I was very confused, wondering if I made a mistake in coming to Italy. I decided to talk about my master, showed pictures, and shared the story of meeting him and studying with him. And believe it or not, something of a miracle happened. I spoke for about one and a half hours, then stopped talking, and waited. Then one person raised her hand and asked, 'When can I show you my pulse?'"

Dr. Naram asked, "How many of you want me to check your pulse?" Most people in the room raised their hands, much to the surprise of both Dr. Naram and Susi.

"On the first day, sixteen people signed up for a pulse healing consultation. The second day, these people told others, so there were thirty-two people waiting. The third day, it had doubled to sixty-four."

Dr. Naram said he was supposed to be in Italy for only two days, but he wound up staying for six, and even that was not enough time to see everyone. So they invited him to come again and speak in other cities.

"That was several decades ago. Since then, I have seen thousands of people here. There are many doctors I have trained, like Dr. Giovanni, Dr. Lisciani, Dr. Chiromaestro, Dr. Lidiana, Dr. Alberto, Dr. Antonella, Dr. Catia, Dr. Guido, and Claudio. So many people's lives have changed for the better. They are healthier and happier."

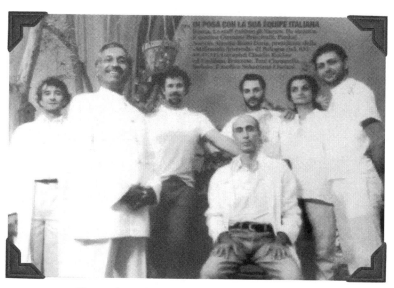

Picture from Oggi *magazine of Dr. Naram and many Italian doctors he was training.*

Dr. Naram told me about Alexander from Germany, who travelled to Italy to meet him. Alexander brought others with him. Soon they had to rent a bus, until finally Dr. Naram accepted Alexander's invitation to come to Germany. Then came invitations to France, Switzerland, Austria, Holland, United Kingdom, the United States, Canada, and many other countries.

"When my master helped me discover that my mission was to bring this ancient healing system into every home, every heart on earth, I didn't believe it. At that time, I didn't even have one

*"My mission is to
bring this ancient
healing system into
every home,
every heart."*

–Dr. Naram

patient. But when this movement of deeper healing started happening in Europe, I was hopeful that my master saw something I didn't. And it just continues. This silent revolution of deeper healing has caught a spark that is now turning into a fire."

Susi stepped in. "Dr. Naram teaches you how to take care of your body before you get sick—how to eat the right food, which herbal supplements to take, and what lifestyle to follow: proper sleeping, exercise, work routines, and how to make time for prayer or meditation. If you know what to do and what not to do, you won't get sick in the first place. This is the real power of Siddha-Veda."

Dr. Naram said, "Susi revealed to you some very important secrets. Yesterday you asked how I have helped women get their periods back, or what I gave to couple's in their eighties to get their vibrant youth back, correct?"

I nodded.

"She just told you how! My master taught me how these things and many more things are possible, through Siddha-Veda's six secret keys to deeper healing. Do you know what the six keys are now?"

I started to get nervous, wondering if this was another test.

"You told me about home remedies, herbal remedies, and marmaa." I said.

"And what are the other three?"

Luckily Susi was overexcited to share them again so I didn't have to guess, "diet, panchakarma or asthakarma, and lifestyle."

Dr. Naram continued, "These powerful ancient healing keys are used by our Siddha-Veda lineage, our 'school of thought', in order to produce results that look to the modern world like miracles. But they are based on time-tested principles and processes, and they produce predictable, long-term, nontoxic results. These keys helped my master live to 125 years young. They are not about a quick fix but rather about a deeper healing."

I found it fascinating that one of his core keys of healing was diet. "But how is diet a 'secret'?" I asked. "Everyone eats food."

Susi said, "Perhaps it's one of those 'secrets' that is right in front of you all the time and you don't notice it until someone points it out."

Dr. Naram added, "Yes, all people eat food. But they usually do not know which foods produce vibrant health, unlimited energy, and peace of mind, and which foods diminish your health, drain your energy, and bring you fear and negative emotions. Do you know which foods can be medicine for one body and yet are poison for another? Do you know which foods nurture your brain, increase your memory power, and foster positive emotions?"

I shook my head *no* to each questions and he continued, "Do you know what times of day are best to eat, and how much to eat, or which foods you should combine together and which you should not? Do you know which foods can keep your immunity strong so you don't get sick, or what foods decrease your *agni* (digestive power) or *bala* (vital energy)? Do you know which foods to avoid when you are overcoming an illness, and which foods help to promote your deeper healing? Knowing these secrets and applying them can help someone have a period again after menopause, overcome hepatitis, nourish kidneys, support an autistic child to become better, or remain vigorously young even in their eighties!"

"There are so many different philosophies on food," I said. "How do I know who is right?"

"Clint, my master taught me this secret. Do not worry about who is right. Only focus on what works."

Susi added, "Yes, there are lots of different theories about what is a healthy diet, what to eat and what not to eat, but there are very few that show these kinds of long-term results in the people who follow them."

Dr. Naram said, "I learned from my master such powerful diet secrets that can change anyone's life. At least they can change the lives of those who want something more than a quick fix for an overall unhealthy lifestyle. These secrets are gold to those who are committed to long-term, nontoxic, deeper healing."

"And what diet secrets did you learn from your master?" I asked.

"Very good question. I wanted to find out what was he doing to live

"If you change your food, you can change your future."

–Dr. Naram

more than a hundred years of age feeling so young? What was he doing differently than most people who start to feel old at fifty? What did he recommend to others that produced such amazing results in their lives, which they weren't seeing from 'quick-fix methods'? One of the biggest differences, he taught me, was in our food."

"Yes, but what did he teach you about food?"

Dr. Naram looked straight at me. "He taught me, if you change your food, you can change your future."

It was a powerful statement. I wanted to change the future for myself and my dad, but wasn't sure what foods we needed to change. "Yes," I said, "I believe you. But what exactly should I eat, and what should I avoid?"

"That is a billion-euro question," Dr. Naram said as he finished his soup and walked slowly to the door. "I need to go back to seeing people now, but I'm very glad you are asking that question. If you learn properly which foods to eat and which to avoid, it can change your life. You will gain a power to know what makes you sick, what makes you healthy, what helps heal you deeply, and what can help you live past one hundred with vibrant health, unlimited energy and peace of mind."

"Please, Dr. Naram, tell me. What do I need to do?"

"Come tomorrow."

And with that he walked out of the room to go back to seeing patients.

Really? I thought. Susi and her mother were also getting called back to the clinic area to help, and I was left alone with my thoughts.

I reflected on recent conversations with my father. Even before going to India, he made some big changes in his diet based on Dr. Naram's recommendations. For most of his life, my dad's typical diet was cereal and milk or bacon and eggs for breakfast. For lunch, he ate cheese sandwiches on wheat bread and potato chips. For dinner, he ate meat and potatoes with a glass of milk. These were the exact foods Dr. Naram recommended avoiding. At first my dad wondered what he *could* eat, but he soon changed his diet from scratch. He stopped eating wheat and dairy products and almost all meat, and started eating cooked green, leafy vegetables and lots of moong bean soup.

Although daunting at first, he soon found satisfaction in alternatives he never considered before. Thankfully, he discovered that there was a huge variety of tasty, healthy foods he never knew existed, many of which were easy to prepare. My dad found substitutes for his old favorite foods, and new recipes he genuinely enjoyed. At the top was Dr. Naram's secret recipe for moong soup. It was rich in protein, reduced inflammation, supplied lots of energy, and still gave him a feeling of lightness. We also learned that the same digestion process needed to metabolize the moong helped the body remove unwanted toxins. All of Dr. Naram's masters living to over one hundred years of age ate moong and lots of ghee. He had given my dad a recipe from the ancient masters for making delicious ghee. Dr. Naram called ghee "magical" because it is so effective at helping balance any of the three dosha types.

My Journal Notes

Dr. Naram's Marvelous Moong Soup Recipe*

Healing Benefits of Moong Beans (sometimes spelled Mung): nutritious, with detoxifying effects, it helps balance all 3 *doshas* (life elements). Aids the clearing away of *aam* (toxicity) that get lodged in the body over time due to poor diet, lack of exercise, and living a sedentary lifestyle.

Many of these ingredients may be purchased online or in Asian/Indian food stores.

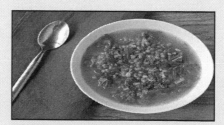

Ingredients:

o 1 cup whole green dried moong beans—soaked overnight
o 2 cups water + 1½ tsp. salt
o 1 Tbs. pure cow's ghee or sunflower oil
o 1 tsp. black mustard seeds
o 2 pinches hing (called asafoetida in the West)
o 1 bay leaf
o ½ tsp. turmeric powder
o 1 tsp. cumin powder
o 1 tsp. coriander powder
o 1 pinch black pepper
o 1½ tsp. fresh ginger, finely chopped
o ½-1 tsp. or 1 clove fresh garlic, finely chopped
o 2 more cups water – add to make the soup after beans are cooked
o 3 pieces of Kokum (dry jungle plum)
o Salt to taste when served

Optional: 1 cup chopped peeled carrots, 1 cup diced celery

PREPARATION STEPS:

1. Rinse, remove any debris, and then soak the moong beans in water overnight. (Add 1 tsp baking soda while it soaks to help reduce gas.)

2. Drain and rinse the moong beans, adding the indicated amount of water and salt, then cook in a pressure cooker until tender. It takes around 25 minutes, depending on your pressure cooker. (The beans have to be broken.)

3. Or, in a regular deep pot, it will take 40-45 minutes for the beans to be fully cooked. Bring to a boil then to low heat with the lid on or cracked slightly. Add Kokum, carrots and celery after 25 minutes.

4. While beans are cooking, after about 20 minutes, heat the oil or ghee in a separate deep pot on medium heat until melted. Add mustard seeds.

5. When the seeds start to pop, add the hing, bay leaf, turmeric, cumin, coriander, ginger, garlic, and a pinch of black pepper and stir gently, mixing well.

6. Quickly turn heat to lowest setting. Simmer about 10 minutes – do not allow to burn.

7. Transfer the cooked beans with 2 more cups fresh water into the pot with the simmering ingredients.

8. Bring to a boil then simmer 5-10 minutes more. Enjoy! May be served with basmati rice.

*Bonus Material: To see how to make this moong soup recipe multiple different delicious ways, as well as to receive other tasty recipes and diet secrets, please refer to the free MyAncientSecrets.com membership site.

Wait, What Do You Mean, "No Pizza"?

Although I enjoyed hearing Susi's experiences, my mind tripped over the part where she said Dr. Naram recommended people stop eating pizza, pasta, cheese, wheat, and milk products. I loved that stuff. What would life be like without pizza? And what about gelato? Why did Dr. Naram think these foods were a problem?

I did some research and learned of the works of Dr. Joel Fuhrman, Dr. Baxter Montgomery, and several other American and European doctors. Their studies answered some of my questions. They revealed a growing body of undeniable evidence regarding the benefits of a plant-based diet. For example, some of their research documented the impact of a plant-based diet on people with severe heart problems and blocked arteries. Western doctors typically insert a stent to push open the vessel, or surgically create a bypass around the block. My dad already had two stents and multiple recommendations for bypass surgery. By changing to a plant-based diet and exercising more, research showed, people could reduce the amount of plaque in their arteries and, in some cases, eliminate it completely.

Dr. Naram had said, "If you change your food, you can change your future."

Could it be that food had such a big impact on our lives? Does what we put in our mouths have that much influence on our health? The connection may seem obvious for others, but it was new to me.

Can the Food You Eat Improve Your Memory?

At one of the clinics in Italy, I met a lawyer named Steven who suffered from skin allergies and asthma. He told me that his mom, dad, and brother were all medical doctors, so he thought they'd have a solution to his problems. Unfortunately, they couldn't find a way to help him. Everything they tried had terrible side effects. Dr. Naram was the first to help him understand that his asthma began not in the lungs, but in his digestion. Steven learned what to eat and what to avoid, and which home remedies and herbal supplements to take. He said his entire life changed once the skin allergies and asthma disappeared. It was an extra bonus that his memory improved, too.

"When I met Dr. Naram," Steven said, "I was in my first year of law school and studying thick and complicated legal books, with thousands of papers to read. It was difficult to focus. Dr. Naram gave me diet recommendations and particular remedies to help improve my memory, and I was able to understand and remember much better than before. My test scores improved. My brain calmed down, making it easier to focus and retain information, which helped me progress at the university."

Steven noted, "Dr. Naram's memory is amazing, too. He remembers what I told him all those years ago, even though he's seen thousands of patients since then. I see him and the way he looks, the way his mind works. It's like time isn't passing for him at all!"

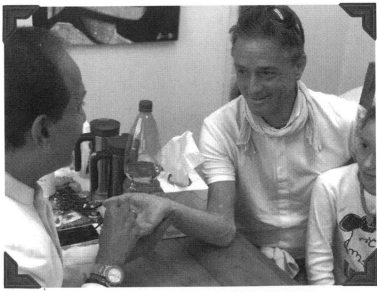

Steven having his pulse taken by Dr. Naram.

My Journal Notes

Additional Ancient Healing Secrets for Improving Your Memory*

Marmaa Shakti—At the base of the outside of your left thumb, press this point 6 times, many times a day.

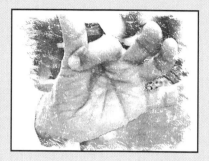

*Bonus Material: To see the marmaa demonstrated, and for more memory secrets, please refer to the free MyAncientSecrets.com membership site.

Steven confided in me that sometimes he didn't follow the diet recommendations completely, but that he was grateful to know that, when he felt ill, he knew the cause and how to reverse it. He said when he didn't know, he didn't even have a choice to be healthy. Now he had a choice.

Food Secrets Most Masters Won't Tell You

Just when I thought I was starting to understand the relationship between diet and health, Dr. Naram scrambled my brain. During his break, with the excitement of a child about to meet Santa, he said "Come with me and Dr. Giovanni, Clint! I must take you somewhere!"

"Where?" I asked.

"For the best pizza in all of Italy!"

When I challenged him about eating pizza, he smiled. "My master told me never to become so emotionally rigid that I become dry. Pizza is not good for my body, true. But it is very good for my emotions. So the question is, how can we occasionally enjoy this food but not at the expense of our health?"

That sounded like a good question to me. I listened intently.

"If you eat these foods every day or even every week, they create toxins in your body and are not good for your digestion. Then you have to go for a long period of not eating them so your body can purify and rebalance. I follow a very strict diet for the whole year, but once a year when I am in Italy I want to enjoy the best pizza. So I prepare my digestion for days beforehand and afterwards, by eating only moong soup and taking herbs that help me digest and not build up toxins. That way I can have food for my emotions and my body doesn't suffer."

He knew exactly which restaurant he wanted to go to. After more than twenty years of coming to Italy, he determined, according to his taste buds, which place had "the best pizza in the world" and which had the most delicious gelato. As we enjoyed our food, he wanted to make sure I understood that when people were overcoming an illness, like his mother or my father, they couldn't digest things like this. It was imperative for them to be disciplined about eating foods that were healthy for them.

He explained how our bodies have a buffer zone that wears down over time. Although eating junk food for years may not seem to have an impact on young bodies, one day, when we are thirty or forty or fifty, something goes wrong. People think it's simply an irreversible process of aging that can be managed only with medications, the side effects of which can lead to other illnesses, requiring more medications. These issues are actually not caused by aging but by the buildup of *aam*, or toxins, from food and the environment, which eventually cause inflammation, blocks, and imbalances.

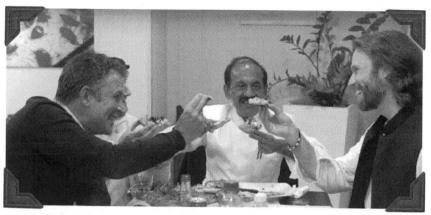

Dr. Naram explained how and when you can even enjoy things like pizza.

Dr. Naram put an extra dab of hot sauce on his pizza and took a bite as Dr. Giovanni told me he learned the hard way that the same food that is medicine for one person can be poison for another.

"When I first saw Dr. Naram use hot sauce, I thought it must be because it was a healthy thing to do, so I started using a lot of hot sauce. Soon I was suffering so much. I didn't know that hot sauce was good for him, acting as a medicine because he is predominantly *kapha* (water/earth dosha), but for me, it was like a poison. I already had a lot of *pitta* (fire dosha) in my body, and so the hot sauce pushed it to an overload." He laughed, remembering that painfully learned lesson. I smiled too, thankful he passed it on to me before I made the same mistake.

As I savored the delicious cheese and crispy crust of my slice, I began to grasp Dr. Naram's philosophy: Once people understand the principles of what creates health versus what creates illness and disease, they also need to remember that life must be enjoyed. If you become too rigid and strict, what is the use of living? Dr. Naram's master taught him how to know what you want, achieve what you want, and then enjoy it. That last part—enjoying it—was essential.

I'll never forget how happy Dr. Naram looked while he ate his pizza.

> *"The same food that can be medicine for one person can be poison for another."*
>
> –Dr. Giovanni

Your Journal Notes

To deepen and magnify the benefits you will experience from reading this book, take a few minutes now and answer the following questions for yourself:

Which ways do you feel changing your food could change your future? (If you were to make a positive change in your diet, what might happen differently in your mind, body, emotions, and relationships?)

_____

_____

_____

_____

_____

What other insights, questions, or realizations came to you as you read this chapter?

_____

_____

_____

_____

_____

Bonus Material: For a more detailed guide to Dr. Naram's overall diet recommendations—as well as his secrets on when/how you could very occasionally "cheat" on a diet and not let it negatively impact your health as much—please refer to the free MyAncientSecrets.com membership site.

CHAPTER 12

Ancient Secrets for Helping Animals, Too?

Those who teach us the most about love aren't always human.
–Author Unknown

As Dr. Giovanni spent much of his day translating for Dr. Naram, he and I met up late one night. After everyone was gone, I asked how he'd come to work with Dr. Naram.

Dr. Giovanni's medical degree is from the University of Bologna (which, as a side-note, has nothing to do with the processed meat I ate as a kid, but is in fact the oldest medical school in Europe). I wanted to know what drew a brilliant medical doctor like him to study an ancient Indian form of treatment for more than seventeen years.

Dr. Giovanni told me it was simple. The solutions allopathic medicine offered left him unsatisfied and wanting more, so he started searching for alternative medicines and treatments. He heard about Dr. Naram during a trip to India in 1984, and knew immediately that he found something extraordinary.

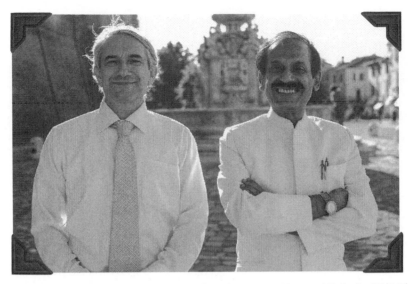

Dr. Naram with one of his most beloved students, Dr. Giovanni Brincivalli, MD.

"When I began studying with Dr. Naram, I used both Western medicine and Siddha-Veda together. I conducted my own research, with the support of a professor from my medical school, on the use of these ancient methods for cases of extreme anxiety and depression. After a few years of studying with Dr. Naram and seeing amazing results, I started using this ancient science exclusively with all my patients."

"How do you feel it affected your medical practice?" I asked.

"For one thing, I never need to prescribe antibiotics or anti-inflammatory drugs anymore. I see the same cases that any family practice doctor sees, and I still am able to use only the deeper healing secrets that I learned from Dr. Naram. The results I get are very, very powerful. People bring their animals, too, and the secrets Dr. Naram taught me also work for them. I am surprised now when I don't see results. But then I talk with Dr. Naram, and he finds something in the ancient manuscripts that helps even in the rarest cases."

Dr. Giovanni currently worked in over twenty cities in Italy. "People come to me for different reasons. It brings me so much satisfaction, so much peace, to have solutions for them."

He described what it was like to work in a psychiatric hospital in Italy. "I was distraught when I'd see patients who were depressed, suicidal, schizophrenic, or had homicidal tendencies locked in rooms. Sometimes they were restrained by chains so they wouldn't hurt themselves or others. They were drugged to suppress the problem and walked around like zombies, with no hope for improvement. When they went to the toilet and the restraining chains were taken off, there'd be two big, burly guards overseeing them to make sure they didn't try to run away. Very difficult to watch."

Dr. Giovanni described his interest in a desperate family who brought their schizophrenic daughter to Dr. Naram. After seeing cases like hers in the hospital, he was curious how Dr. Naram would approach her treatment. "When they first came, the parents had her on strong medication to keep her calm and controlled. She was sluggish and lethargic and had sudden mood swings. For example, she would suddenly grab and rip up any papers she found on the table."

After six months of Dr. Naram's treatment, her situation changed dramatically. Her medication was reduced by half, and she started smiling more. She was more conscious and alert, more present and joyful.

"We never saw or even expected such an improvement in the hospital setting. What also impressed me was how much it changed the quality of life for the entire family. This was inspiring. When I asked Dr. Naram how this worked, he told me that ninety percent of our problems come from emotional wounds or trauma from childhood. Then he taught me the ancient methods to help heal these wounds, and over the last seventeen years, I've seen them work over and over again, in even the most extreme cases."

Again, my thoughts went to my sister, who had struggled with depression and eventually took her own life. I wasn't ready to talk with Dr. Giovanni about it, but I wondered whether Dr. Naram would have been able to help her. All doctors could do at the time was give her medications that didn't work.

Dr. Giovanni described another case he saw early on with Dr.

"Ninety percent of our problems come from emotional wounds or trauma from childhood."

–Dr. Naram

Naram that left a deep impression on him. A man who had three major arterial blockages in his heart was suffering from shortness of breath and could walk only a few steps without pain in his chest. "I studied this topic in medical school. According to Western medicine, there is no good way to reverse arterial blocks. We can only insert a stent and enlarge the blood vessel or create a cardiac bypass. The cardiologists told this man to go immediately for surgery because he was at high risk for a massive heart attack. The man refused and came to Dr. Naram. After he followed Dr. Naram's advice for three and a half months, his disposition and subsequent tests showed the blocks were reversing." Dr. Giovanni's voice revealed how impressed he was by this result.

"I was inspired," Dr. Giovanni recalled, "as I never thought this was possible. This man went through a powerful, ancient process of deeper healing. He did panchakarma, took herbal remedies, and followed a prescribed diet. He took responsibility for his life, changed his habits, and ate lots of moong and vegetables."

Dr. Giovanni looked at me and said, "I am proud of you that you have an open mind to learn all about this."

All Dogs Go to Heaven, but Why Go Sooner than Necessary?

Feeling more open to express my ever-nagging doubts, I asked Dr. Giovanni, "Do you think there's any possibility there could be a placebo effect? That because people strongly believe the diet or remedies will work, they suddenly feel better?"

Dr. Giovanni said, "Good question, Clint. First, look at Rabbat, who was in a coma and got better. How could that have been placebo? Then look at how Dr. Naram also helps animals. I've seen him treat many animals, including tigers, elephants, dogs, horses, owls, kangaroos, crocodiles, and cats. Do animals believe they will get better? Yet the ancient methods heal them, too. Through his foundation, Dr. Naram sponsors many animal shelters, in which they also use the natural herbal remedies to help the street dogs and other wounded or sick animals. Did you meet Paula today?"

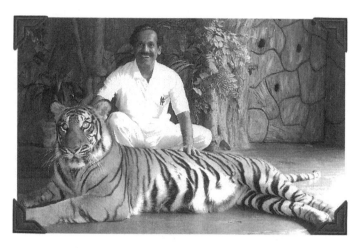

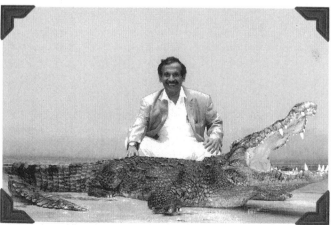

Top: This Royal Bengal tiger could not get pregnant until Dr. Naram felt her pulse and gave certain herbs and diet, and soon she had three babies.
Bottom: This crocodile was angry, and the zoo didn't know why . . .
Through the pulse Dr. Naram discovered it was a constipation problem,
and after being given the right herbs the crocodile was happy again!

"Yes," I responded.

Earlier in the day I was surprised when a sixty-four-year-old woman named Paula arrived with her two dogs. She was very emotional as she told me that years ago one of her dogs, a black Labrador, was sick and in so much pain that he couldn't walk. The veterinarian couldn't help, and she was about to put him to sleep. Paula didn't know how she could handle the agony of knowing she chose to kill her beloved dog. He was in so much pain she did not know what else to do. While she was jogging that morning, she found out from a friend that Dr. Naram was in Italy. She promptly went home, loaded her dog in the car, and drove across the country to meet him.

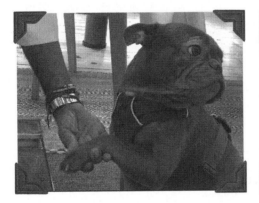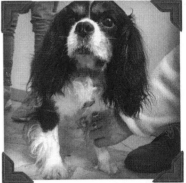

Dr. Naram & Dr. Giovanni taking the pulse of dogs.

"I was desperate," Paula told me. "Dr. Naram took his pulse and told me exactly what was wrong: my dog was full of *aam* (toxins) and had osteoporosis. I did everything he told me to do. I gave him the special herbal formulas and restricted diet, and after only one week, he jumped in the car again! He jumped! He didn't limp anymore, and for three more years he was perfect. Perhaps because animals don't think the same as people, I feel they are much purer. Maybe the remedies work faster for them than in people. I don't know, but that's what happened. Even when he grew older, he was still strong and healthy until he passed away peacefully at home."

Helping Bees?

Dr. Giovanni went on to tell me another story about a friend of his who was a beekeeper. A destructive parasite infected her bees with a virus and they stopped producing honey and started dying. To kill the parasites, other beekeepers chose to expose the bees to poisonous fumes, which unfortunately also killed a lot of bees. Those that survived were full of chemicals that impacted the quality of their honey. Because they ate the honey and also planned to sell it, the woman and her family wanted to choose a nonchemical solution. They called Dr. Giovanni.

"I went to see the bees and at first, had no clue how to help them," he explained. "How do you catch the pulse of bees without getting stung?" He smiled, and I laughed at the image in my head of him trying to find the pulse of a bee. Dr. Giovanni showed me the marmaa point for boosting immunity in humans, then asked me, "But how do you do this for the bees?"

My Journal Notes

Ancient Healing Secrets for Boosting Immunity*

Marmaa Shakti—On the right hand, middle finger very top portion, press 6 times, many times a day.

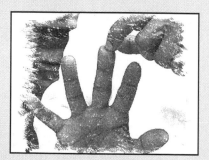

*Bonus Material: For a powerful home remedy that helped boost their immunity to overcome the virus, please see the appendix and visit the free membership site.

"I did some research and learned that this kind of infection makes the bees weak. They don't fly, and some lose all their body hair. Healthy bees start fighting with the sick bees, as they don't recognize them as their own. This gave me an idea."

Dr. Giovanni remembered a story of Dr. Naram growing his own hair back. He also discovered which herbs boost immunity. He and the beekeeper crushed some of Dr. Naram's herbal tablets designed to boost immunity and grow hair, mixed them with a powerful home remedy that included honey, and fed it to the bees.

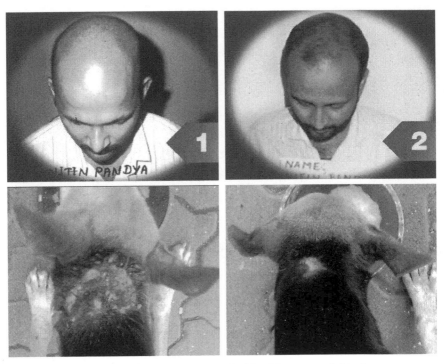

Knowing Dr. Naram helped many people, like this man and this dog, to grow their hair back, Dr. Giovanni used this as part of the way to also help the bees.

A short time later Dr. Giovanni got a call from the beekeeper. "The bees are growing their hair back! And they look stronger, healthier." Slowly, the population of bees increased and they were producing an abundance of honey. To honor the moment and the special honey the bees made, they called it "Ancient Secrets

Honey." The beekeeper believed the nonchemical honey reflected the properties of immunity and stamina from the herbal remedies they gave the bees.

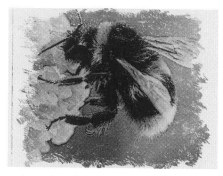

Even bees have been helped with the ancient healing secrets.

When I discussed this with Dr. Naram later, he told me, "Believe it or not, these ancient healing secrets work on human beings, animals, and also plants. Because we are all a part of nature, the same principles apply."

The story touched me, as I had seen reports in the news of bee populations around the world dwindling, with sobering questions about the long-term impacts on global sustainability if these pollinators disappeared. If only more people like Dr. Giovanni were studying and using these practices.*

"What advice do you have for others who want to learn this method of ancient healing?"

"It is a constant process, Clint." Dr. Giovanni said. "You need an open heart and mind. If you simply want to learn things that can help you, that is very possible. Anyone on this planet can learn ancient secrets that will change their life if they commit to diligently follow them. But to become a healer requires inner development, not just technical knowledge. Dr. Naram says to be a true healer is not just about knowing, but about doing, and most importantly about your being. When you work with animals, too, they can especially feel your being. To achieve the state of being of a master healer, you must dedicate your life."

> "Ancient healing secrets work on human beings, animals, and also plants."
> –Dr. Naram

Bonus Material: To discover more about ancient secrets for communicating with animals, as well as secrets for having healthy full hair, please refer to the free MyAncientSecrets.com membership site.

"To become a true healer requires inner development, not just technical knowledge."

–Dr. Giovanni

He explained the tricky part for anyone is that most people are addicted to their habits. "For example, in Italy, everyone thinks a 'good diet' is pasta, cheese, and wine. Then, when they become ill they want a quick fix with some pills. That is their choice. But at what cost? There are serious, long-term side effects of those pills. As an alternative, when people choose the path of deeper healing, they need to pay the price of some discipline to change their habits, patience, persistence, and determination. As a result, they experience long-term deeper healing and peace of mind. It's just a choice. What price are you willing to pay?"

Dr. Giovanni paused so I could take in what he was sharing. I could see what he meant with people I'd seen, including my father.

"What inspires people to choose to change their habits, their life, so they can experience deeper healing? At first, they need faith or confidence in the healer to follow their advice long enough to feel the difference. After they begin seeing results, they continue for a long time and share it with others. This choice of deeper healing is profound. For most, it requires a lasting change in perspective, which is often hard to do."

His words made me reflect on my father and some of our recent conversations. Our ideas were changing about things as basic as which foods were good for us. For my dad to do an extensive detoxification treatment in India was a major change. *Ultimately*, I still wondered, *would these changes make enough of a difference in such an extreme case as my father?* There was a lot at stake. My dad invested significant money, time, effort, and hope into restructuring his life so he could accommodate every recommendation Dr. Naram gave him. My fear was that if it didn't work, he might become more depressed and discouraged than before and return to preparing for his own death.

Talking to those who benefited from Dr. Naram's approach gave me more confidence that this was a trusted ancient system that worked. But would it work for *my* dad?

Unusual Update from My Father

One day I took a walk through the city center of Milan. I was pleased to discover I could pick up free Wi-Fi on my phone. As I opened my email, I saw that I had received an update from my dad.

August 3, 2010 — Day 3 Report

It is 7:15 p.m. in Mumbai, 6:45 a.m. in Utah. I am at the end of my second day of treatment, getting better adjusted and feeling a little more comfortable in the very different living conditions in Mumbai as opposed to Salt Lake City. My diet today consisted of a plate of sliced papaya for breakfast and a bowl of moong bean soup for lunch and dinner. The day's activities consisted of yoga from 7:30 a.m. to 8:30 a.m., meeting with Dr. Swapna, one of the great doctors here at the Ayushakti clinic, and another full massage with a warm, grainy substance that left me feeling vigorously scrubbed. I imagine it is much like a car feels after emerging from a car wash; except after the rubdown, you are left coated with a substance that you are not to wash off for three to four hours. I have yet to take my cold shower for the day. Beyond that, I was able to consume the twenty different herbal remedies I'm taking both in the morning and in the evening. As a result, most of the abdominal and chest pains I've been experiencing appear to have gone away—I guess there is not much in moong bean soup and sliced papaya to offend the digestive system. Actually, the food is pleasant and I haven't seemed to want much more, so the quantity is sufficient. The restaurant will serve me all I want, but that is all I have wanted today.

I read his email as I sat under the arch of a sprawling fountain in the middle of an open square. My dad was doing yoga? I smiled at the thought. I smiled even bigger hearing he was beginning to feel different.

He also said one of his favorite parts was meeting interesting people at the clinic from Kenya, England, Germany, and elsewhere. One case that left a big impression on him was a woman who had multiple sclerosis and was unable to walk for twenty years. With Dr. Naram's help, she lost over fifty pounds and now was able to hold a job working for the Red Cross in Germany. Her dream in coming to India was to get her body in good enough condition that she could walk again. My dad described the emotion of watching her take her first steps.

Later that night, I reached my dad on Skype to hear more. He told me that when he started the treatments, his body was so tender that the massages were uncomfortable. When I asked him if he was enjoying it, he laughed, saying, "I'm not sure 'enjoying' is the right word, but I'm grateful for it."

He explained that the first stages of the treatment were designed to take toxins out of his body, which took time and patience. The next steps were to help build his body back up again.

Even if my dad didn't feel great yet, being with the other patients and hearing their stories comforted him. Having good, healthy food and a semi-predictable routine made things easier, too. Overall, he sounded hopeful. Feeling him more settled helped me shed some concerns and feel more relaxed.

With good news from my dad and all the stories Dr. Giovanni and others shared with me that day swimming in my head, I wondered again why more people didn't know about the deeper healing options of Siddha-Veda.

By now I had met so many people (and animals) whose lives were changed due to Dr. Naram and his work. I reflected on how I was changing, too. My state of being was shifting into a more grounded, peaceful place inside me. I didn't know how or why, but

I was feeling better about myself and life in general. My questions were changing from "Does this work?" to "How does this work?" and from "How can anyone believe in this stuff?" to "Why don't more people know this exists?"

With so much evidence, the skeptic in me was less visible as I became more hopeful this really was a solid, predictable approach to healing. And if that was the case, why was it so difficult for people to choose to follow it? Why is it such a challenge to make changes that benefit our health? Why did most of the people who came to Dr. Naram have to reach a point of desperation before realizing there was a healthier, better way to live? And why were unhealthy habits so hard to break?

Your Journal Notes

To deepen and magnify the benefits you will experience from reading this book, take a few minutes now and answer the following questions for yourself:

What old wounds do you have that are still likely affecting you today?

_____

_____

_____

What old habits are you "addicted" to which are likely holding you back from what you want most?

_____

_____

_____

What wisdom do you feel we can learn from animals, insects, and/or plants?

_____

_____

_____

What other insights, questions, or realizations came to you as you read this chapter?

_____

_____

_____

CHAPTER 13

Lessons from History: Greatest Obstacles and Greatest Discoveries

*A simple paradigm shift is all it takes to
change the course of your life forever.*

–Jeff Spires

Wanting answers, during my remaining time in Milan, I reached out to two people. The first was my friend Dr. John Rutgers, who received a medical degree but also studied many forms of alternative and complementary medicine. I had met him years earlier and heard him share several remarkable healing experiences with alternative medicine.

Back then, I enjoyed being with John, but to be honest, I thought his perspectives seemed a bit . . . well, eccentric. Now, I had to admit that my own views about health limited my options, as I would minimize any opinions that didn't fit the mainstream. Since meeting Dr. Naram, my perspective was widening. My so-called eccentric friend John suddenly seemed like someone whose valuable insights I had simply not been ready to hear. I felt he could help me understand some things and asked if he had time for a Skype call.

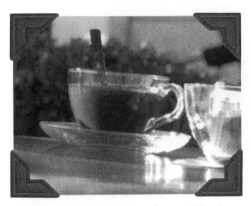

Thick Italian hot chocolate ... Yum!

To assure a strong internet connection, I found a café in a quaint part of the city that had not only great Wi-Fi but also thick hot chocolate with the consistency of a melted chocolate bar. I loved it. With my internet connection and Italian hot chocolate in place, I told John some of the things I saw and heard at Dr. Naram's clinics in India, California, and Italy. He was genuinely interested and I appreciated his sincere engagement with my flood of doubts and questions.

"Why, with all the money spent in American medical research universities, have they not yet discovered how to do what Dr. Naram is doing? If this kind of healing is possible and these people are seeing life-altering results, why don't more know about this kind of medicine? Why is there resistance to it?"

John paused for a long moment. "Let's start with the big picture. Since the beginning of humanity, mankind has been trying to find ways to explain what seemed out of our control—storms, changes in seasons, famine, as well as sickness and disease. Events that impacted human lives and crop production created a big need to find order. That allowed us to have more control over the outcome of these events, which in turn increased our chance of survival. Does that make sense to you?"

"I guess so."

"Take ancient civilizations. They looked up and saw the stars and planets in the night sky, moving in a way they couldn't explain. They came to think of them as gods that controlled the elements on earth, like the weather or someone's health, based on their moods. They created stories around these heavenly bodies to explain otherwise inexplicable events, which helped give meaning to the world around them.

"Effectively, it's the same impulse as science," John continued. "While science and religion sometimes seem at odds with each other, they are actually expressions of the same thing: a desire for order in our lives."

When I was growing up, faith played a big part in my life, and then as a university researcher I shifted my focus to science. Although I never personally felt science and faith conflicted, though I've certainly known those who did, I never considered this idea that they were in the same realm.

John then added, "Once we humans find a belief that gives our minds a sense of order, meaning, and predictability and we find security in that belief, it becomes difficult to change, no matter what evidence we have to the contrary. We gather as much evidence as we can to reinforce our belief, and at the same time, we ignore, fear, or reject any evidence that challenges it. For example, how often do people visit a church that is not their own or read a book by someone with a political viewpoint that challenges theirs?"

"Not often," I admitted.

"Exactly. The human brain fears disorder and uncertainty, so it tries to resist them to maintain order. And we limit ourselves by this tendency and it becomes an obstacle to seeing new ideas that we may benefit from. Take the case of Galileo—he was Italian. Do you know much about his story?"

I looked out the café window, across the charming Italian street and saw clothes hanging out to dry between the buildings. "Wasn't Galileo known for his discovery that the Earth revolves around the sun, and not the other way around?"

"Actually, it was Copernicus who used mathematics to discover this in the 1500s, but nobody paid much attention at that point. Eighteen hundred years prior to Copernicus, the Greek philosopher Aristotle challenged the notion that the planets and stars were just gods wandering around. Instead, he proposed that they were objects or spheres that rotated in a fixed path around the Earth, which people accepted. In 1609, Galileo used the telescope to look at the night sky and concluded that Copernicus was right: not everything revolved around the Earth."

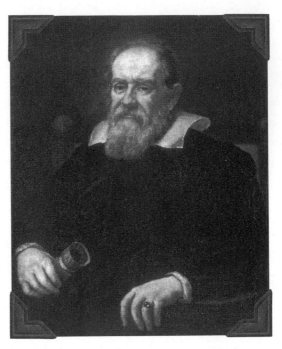

Portrait of Galileo Galilei, Justus Sustermans, 1636. Retrieved from Wikimedia.

Gazing at the street, I wondered what this neighborhood in Milan would have looked like in the 1600s. The cobblestone streets and ancient-looking buildings made it easy to imagine. John continued, "Galileo published his findings in Italian and not the usual Latin, so the masses could read it. Latin was accessible *only* to academics. He provided evidence that the previous belief about the Earth was incorrect. With a more accurate understanding of the solar system, much could be improved, including the calendar, understanding of seasons, and so on. So how do you think people responded?"

"I think people found it hard to accept," I said. "I remember learning in school that the pope at the time condemned him to house arrest, right?" I reflected on what Dr. Giovanni said: that when a new viewpoint is presented, it is difficult for people to change perspectives.

"Yes. Why do you think academicians, the church, the scientific establishment of his day, and even the pope would be so concerned about Galileo challenging the idea that the Earth was the center of the universe?"

Finishing the last of my hot chocolate, I tried to figure out why they would take such a stance. "I don't know," I said. "Why?"

"Partly because the human brain resists disorder. In this case, people were afraid of an idea that contradicted something that seemed certain. It's what researchers call 'confirmation bias,' and it's one of the worst mistakes we can ever make—to discount something too early because it goes against what we think we already know."

"I get that," I said, sharing my initial resistance to Dr. Naram and his work. "In fact, I'm still struggling, which was why I called you."

"Look," said John. "It's not that people will never accept what Dr. Naram is doing. Actually, more and more medical doctors are discovering the benefits of things like meditation, yoga, and plant-based diets. But the mainstream hasn't accepted it yet, as it takes time and money to do research and disseminate findings. Especially because the paradigms of the Western scientific model don't know how to make sense of or even measure the impact of these traditional ancient healing sciences."

"What do you mean about paradigms?" I asked.

"Let's say you're playing football, and a bunch of baseball players come over and tell you that you're not playing a real sport because you're not adhering to the rules of sports. To qualify their statement, they point out you're not using a bat, and the ball is too big and the wrong shape. The truth is that you are just not adhering to the rules of baseball. Likewise, the Western scientific and medical paradigm has certain fixed assumptions that allow it to see in certain ways. This led to some great discoveries and yet also blinded it to seeing other things. That doesn't mean that other forms of science or inquiry are not useful. Dr. Naram is not playing the same game Western doctors are, but that doesn't mean that what he is doing isn't valid."

He gave me another analogy, "You can't compare a fish to a bird and say one is better than the other—they do different things. You

"You can't say football is not a sport because it doesn't adhere to the rules of baseball. Dr. Naram is not playing the same game Western doctors are, but that doesn't mean that what he is doing isn't valid."

–Dr. John Rutgers

can't judge a fish by how well it can fly."

"I understand that analogy," I said. "But isn't science beyond culture?"

"Actually sciences, like cultures, come with their own sets of assumptions and rules for what things mean and what counts as important. Like your story about your headache and the onion rings. The Western model would set up an experiment to see if onion rings do indeed help headaches. In a double-blind study, neither doctors nor the patients would know who was getting the placebo (essentially a sugar pill), the proven pain killer, or the new substance—in your case, onion rings. Then they'd see if the patients who received the onion treatment had different results. Does that make sense?"

I nodded.

"And if they can't prove there are significant differences between the onion rings and the placebo, a traditional scientific study would determine that this traditional form of healing isn't effective."

"So you're saying that modern science hasn't shown this stuff is better than placebo?" I asked.

"All this proves is that their methods of testing are not yet effective at revealing the efficacy of healing modalities and procedures outside their own paradigm. Dr. Naram told you there are many different kinds of headaches, and that onions are specifically useful for one of the types. He is personalizing care based on things he can feel in the pulse that modern Western medical equipment is nowhere near able to detect. Whereas Western science often says, 'You have a headache so here's a pill,' it sounds like Dr. Naram distinguishes which type of headache you have, then looks at your particular constitution to draw from a wide variety of remedies."

"You can't compare a fish to a bird and say one is better than the other— they do different things."

–Dr. John Rutgers

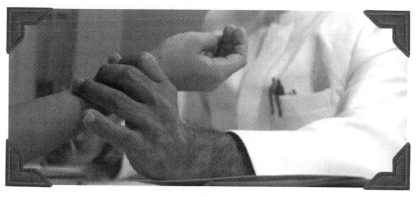

Dr. Naram taking the pulse of someone, by which he can detect subtle imbalances and blocks that impact physical, mental, and emotional well-being.

"Alright," I said, starting to get it, "because Dr. Naram is not treating a disease but personalizing treatment for the whole person, the most common methods of validation in the Western scientific paradigm won't be able to measure it?"

"Right," John said. "But what I'm noticing is that the wisest doctors with brilliant minds and open hearts, those who really want to help people, are coming around. The Hippocratic Oath, to do no harm, is an oath all new doctors take when beginning their career. In light of this oath, many wise doctors see their current methods may be doing harm to patients when compared to the natural ancient remedies, then they become open to other complementary ways of helping

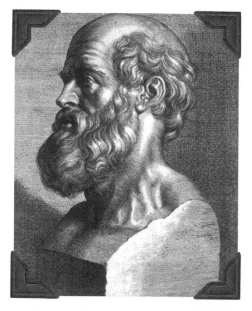

Hippocrates, Greek physician referred to as the "Father of Medicine." Engraving by Peter Paul Rubens, 1638. Shared courtesy of the National Library of Medicine.

and healing. The greatest discoveries are always made by people willing to open up to something new and unfamiliar. Otherwise, most ordinary people resist new beliefs until their other options have failed them."

"That's true," I said. "A lot of people come to Dr. Naram as a last resort, rather than as a way to prevent them from even having whatever illness they're suffering from in the first place—which he says his techniques can do. If that's true, it would save them a lot of trouble and pain to come before the problems start. Why doesn't Western medicine focus more on prevention?"

"Look," said John. "Every culture from the beginning of time has sought out the fountain of youth, wellness, and healing. Shamans, witch doctors, and medicine men and women have always been sought out to help people find solutions to maintaining health or overcoming illness, some more effective than others. It's important to understand how Western medicine came to be 'Western' medicine."

Some noise outside the window prompted me to look up. I saw a group of school children walking by, speaking in animated Italian voices. I focused in again on John as he began sharing a brief and fascinating history of Western medicine as we know it.

"For a long time," he explained, "doctors in the United States practiced a combination of healing models, including naturopathy, homeopathy, hydrotherapy, and Thomsonian medicine, which relied heavily on Native American herbal remedies and sweat baths. Then, in 1910, a study was done to determine which healing approach was most effective. Its findings ultimately resulted in the closure of 120 medical schools, leaving only 32. According to the way they measured things in the report, the best model was found at Johns Hopkins University. It came to be known as 'allopathy,' from Greek roots that meant 'different suffering.' Essentially, it referred to the practice of healing through opposites. If someone has a bad cough, give them a cough suppressant.

"An influx of money from financial backers trying to help standardize medicine in America, combined with the preference for allopathy, created a big shift in policy and regulations. The shift had some positive effects, like the eradication of polio and a decrease in the number of snake-oil salesmen. It also created some significant limitations. It led to the systematic suppression of effective forms of holistic healing that didn't fit the same paradigm."

I never heard any of this before. Shifting in my seat, I challenged what John said. "Look, even with its downsides, our Western medical system is sought after by people all over the world. It must be more effective than other methods."

"Think of it this way," John replied. "If allopathy, the dominant model of medicine at the moment, really is superior in understanding health, wellness, and longevity, then why is the life expectancy of doctors lower than that of the average person? And why is the suicide rate among doctors so high? At the same time, why are so many men, women, and children in Western society becoming more obese and more depressed? Why are we seeing more illness, not less? I agree there are advancements, but it also seems to me that the dominant paradigm is missing something."

Later, reflecting on what John said, I realized how much of what he told me applied to what Dr. Naram was doing. People had their own ideas and philosophies about diet: what was good to eat and what was not, what made them sick, and what to do to stay healthy. Those beliefs gave them a sense of certainty. And when someone challenged those beliefs, it was difficult to change perspective unless they were desperate and *had* to seek something else.

I had much to consider. For years, I believed I was open-minded to other belief systems and loved immersing myself in them during my travels. Now I realized just how fixed my belief systems were. I accepted so many things as true because they were what I was taught. I sincerely believed that America and Europe had the best medical practitioners on the planet. I never considered that our

medical system had blind spots, that it could be missing fundamental components to understanding and promoting health,
wellness, and longevity. I was perplexed. Whom could I trust when
I needed effective healthcare?

While traveling in Mexico, I had met a university professor from
Germany who lived in Toronto named Ludwig Max Fischer (a.k.a.
Max). He spent a good portion of his life researching ancient healing traditions around the world. I was instantly fascinated by his
perspective on issues I struggled to understand. I also reached out
to Max, asking if we could have a call, and he picked up where John
left off.

"Why did you start researching this area?" I asked.

"When I was a young professor, I had a stomach pain that per-
sisted for a year and a half." With a soft German accent, Max's voice
had a warm, soothing quality that made me feel as if I was talking
to a wise grandfather. "I went to doctors throughout Europe and
the United States. They gave me one treatment after another, but
nothing worked—and some of the side effects were awful." It got
so bad, he was bedridden much of the time.

"Out of desperation, I met with a healer from an Eastern tradition. He told me there was an imbalance of the elements in my
system: 'Too much wood in your body,' he said.

"At the time I remember thinking 'He can't be serious! I haven't
eaten any wood.' To my academically trained ears, it sounded
ridiculous.

"Out of desperation, I followed the healer's advice and was
surprised how quickly I got better."

"That's amazing," I said.

"What's amazing," Max replied, "is that although I regained my
health, I had mixed feelings about it. On one hand, I was grateful
the advice worked. On the other hand, I was frustrated. I was too

proud to admit that my Western education had failed me. It took a while to process my feelings, but in my search for truth, I began a lifelong study of ancient healing traditions around the world."

I was captivated by what Max was saying. He continued, "Only later I discovered insights into how that healer analyzed and solved my problem so quickly. I realized that in modern Western medicine, we make everything into a fight. We fight disease, we fight bacteria, we fight cancer. In the Eastern system, and in other ancient traditions, it's not about fighting, but rather creating balance through purification. Great healers of these ancient traditions are adept at identifying imbalances and prescribing remedies to cleanse and rebalance the system."

"If these ancient forms of healing are so effective," I asked, "why do so many respected people minimize or reject them? For example, when I tried telling a friend of mine who's a doctor from America about what I saw in India, he immediately said these herbs and ancient methods are not scientifically proven."

Max listened deeply and thoughtfully replied, "I believe it's arrogant of us in the modern Western system to automatically reject another approach by calling it 'not scientifically proven.' That merely means it doesn't fit our limited and relatively young tradition of 'modern' medical science, which has only been around for a couple hundred years. The concept of 'allopathic' medicine only came into existence in 1810.

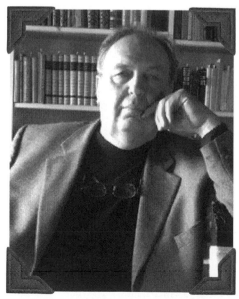

"In contrast, so many of the so-called 'alternative' sciences have been refined by great scholars and healers for thousands of years,

Professor Ludwig Max Fischer, PhD.

taking into account many variables that our scientists haven't yet considered, many of which our instruments can't measure."

While Max spoke, I thought of how Dr. Naram began so many conversations by referring to his unbroken lineage that goes back over 2,500 years. I had to admit that for anything to last that long, it must be doing something right.

"Our perspective is also very reductionistic," Max continued. "By this I mean we break things into parts. For example, Western medicine breaks a person into parts, then focuses only on those parts. We take into consideration only those things we can measure. We rely primarily on the capture of static data regarding those parts, putting it into charts and graphs. And if we don't find what we're looking for, we assume that *absence of evidence* is *evidence of absence*—but it's not!

"By contrast, the ancient healing ways consider the *whole* system. They understand how one part influences all other parts, and how to bring them all into balance."

Max said that some Eastern traditions acknowledge that certain wisdom and knowledge can't be captured in a book, taught in a course, or measured with instruments. It can only be learned and passed down by a direct transmission from a master to an apprentice. It acknowledges that there is power contained in the collective wisdom and experience of masters in a lineage, developed over thousands of years. That certainly seemed to be the case with Dr. Naram and the lineage of healers he became part of.

I thought back to what John said about Dr. Naram not fitting any of the categories that people in the world today relate to. For Dr. Naram, it's not about being ancient or modern, Western or Eastern, homeopathic or allopathic, Ayurvedic or Chinese, or anything else. It's about deeper healing and discovering what works.

"You were curious about Dr. Naram because you saw the results of his approach, right?" Max asked me.

I agreed.

"Most people don't know how electricity works, but when they see a light in the middle of a dark house, they usually walk toward it."

I smiled at the analogy.

"Although people like Dr. Naram are operating via rules and frameworks that most of us don't understand, what we see is his caring and devotion to patients. He is a light that so many people are attracted to in their darkest hours. They may not know how it works, but a burning desire for health guided them to him. There is a Buddhist saying, 'When the student is ready, the teacher appears.' Similarly, I believe that when the patient is open and ready, the healer appears."

> *"Most people don't know how electricity works, but when they see a light in the middle of a dark house, they usually walk toward it. Dr. Naram is a light that so many people are attracted to in their darkest hours. They may not know how it works, but a burning desire for health guided them to him."*
>
> –Dr. Ludwig Max Fischer

Thanks to the conversations with John and Max, I sensed a shift inside me, like tectonic plates readjusting. They helped me understand that Dr. Naram used an actual science, with internally consistent principles that helped him see and solve problems Western medicine didn't yet understand. Although helpful, this realization also challenged me. Could it be that what I accepted to be true my entire life—that Western medicine was the best bet people had to heal themselves in times of illness—was not the absolute truth, but merely a belief I held? Is it possible that our medical system could have blind spots and could be missing components that are fundamental to understanding and promoting health, wellness, and longevity?

Your Journal Notes

To deepen and magnify the benefits you will experience from reading this book, take a few minutes now and answer the following questions for yourself:

What things have you believed in your life that you later discovered were not true?

_____

_____

_____

_____

Can you think of times when you have been ready for something (e.g., a teacher, a healing), and once you were truly ready it suddenly appeared?

_____

_____

_____

_____

What other insights, questions, or realizations came to you as you read this chapter?

CHAPTER 14

_____

_____

_____

_____

Secrets for Discovering Your Life's Purpose

The meaning of life is to find your gift.
The purpose in life is to give it away.
–Pablo Picasso

There is a famous Gothic cathedral in Milan called the Duomo. It is one of the largest cathedrals in Italy, and Dr. Naram likes to visit it every time he's in the city. As Simone, Dr. Naram's country coordinator, drove us through the crowded streets toward the Duomo, I thought about how much and how rapidly my perspective of the world, and of myself, was changing. There was a struggle inside me and I couldn't work out why I felt such a lack of peace and direction.

"Do you remember the three greatest achievements in this life, according to my lineage?" As we sat in the back seat together, Dr. Naram quizzed me again.

I tried to remember. "Let's see. Number one, to know what you want; number two, to achieve what you want; and number three, to enjoy what you have achieved?"

"Correct. Siddha-Veda is a school of thought that helps with these on physical, mental, and emotional levels." He smiled.

"Can I share with you a priceless secret my master shared with me?" Dr. Naram asked. "This one is about discovering and achieving what you want in life. You'll never guess how it happened for me. One day, my master asked me, 'What do you want?' And I said, 'How do I know?' Then he gave me a great gift by showing me the secret marmaa. This is the same marmaa point I pressed on my mother to discover what she wanted."

Dr. Naram's master told him to close his eyes, press the marmaa point on the tip of his right index finger six times, then be silent. After some time, he gave Dr. Naram a series of questions to consider. Dr. Naram emphasized the importance and value of those questions and how much they could change my life.

"These are the billion-dollar questions you can ask yourself to discover your purpose in life:

> If you only had six months to live, what would you most want to do or be?
> If you knew you could not fail, what would you most want to do or be?
> If you had ten million dollars in the bank and never needed to work again, what would you most want to do or be?"

As Simone continued weaving our car through Milan's streets, I wrote the questions down, feeling a familiar discomfort. Even if I allowed myself to ask them, would I have answers? Most days, I had no idea what I wanted to do or be in my life, a sharp contrast to this man, who was intensely focused and present at all times.

Dr. Naram continued, "My answer to my master's question was, 'I would like to be a great healer.' He told me, 'The clearer are the goals, the more certain are the chances.' Then he helped me gain more clarity by painting a specific picture in my mind. He pressed different marmaa points on my finger as he asked me additional questions."

"What do you mean by 'great healer?'" Baba Ramdas asked.

Dr. Naram replied, "I want to be the best pulse healer on this planet, a master of these ancient healing secrets."

> *"The clearer are the goals, the more certain are the chances."*
> –Baba Ramdas
> (Dr. Naram's Master)

His master encouraged him, saying, "Very good, Pankaj. Write it down."

Dr. Naram told me, "Even though some of this desire came from ego and fear, as I wanted to prove to my dad and everyone else that I was worthy, my master didn't challenge or discourage me from dreaming. On the contrary, he encouraged it! He then asked me another difficult question, 'How will you know you are the best?'"

This is when Dr. Naram interrupted his own story, looked at me, and said, "I'm not sharing this with you because of my ego, so please try to understand. It is not about me right now, or impressing you, but about inspiring you to consider what is possible. Since you are asking sincere questions, trying to discover more about your life, I want you to succeed. In 1982, my father kicked me out of our house after a fight. I had less than a dollar in my pocket. I was angry, lonely, confused, frustrated, unhealthy, and depressed. I didn't know where to go and sleep that night. It was thanks to my master that I eventually discovered who I was and what was possible to do with my life."

Dr. Naram said his master continued to question him, asking, "How will you know you are the best pulse healer?"

"When I have seen a hundred thousand people, I will know."

"What else?"

"I will know when people come from six countries to see me."

"Fantastic, now write it down. What else?"

"I will be the best when Mother Teresa comes to me and says, 'Dr. Naram, you are doing the greatest work on this planet.'"

"Very good. What else?"

"I will also know when His Holiness, The Dalai Lama comes and asks me to read his pulse."

My Journal Notes

Additional Marmaa Shakti Secrets for Getting Clarity in What You Want* (Continued from Chapter 9, p.136)

7) On the bottom portion of your pointer finger of your right hand, press this point 6 times.

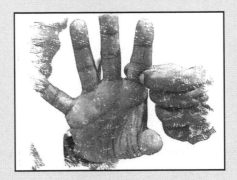

8) Ask yourself, "If I had or became what I want, what exactly would it look like?"

9) Write down the answers that come to you, and keep asking the questions until a clear picture is formed.

*Bonus Material: To have Dr. Naram walk you through this process, please refer to the videos in the free MyAncientSecrets.com membership site.

Dr. Naram paused and said, "All of these desires came into my heart before I had a single patient. I only had a dream. My master was encouraging, but when I told my friends and family, they laughed. They couldn't see why so many people would want to come see me, or why the Dalai Lama or Mother Teresa would be interested in my pulse healing."

"When someone has a dream, support them. Don't sabotage them," Dr. Naram said. "I almost gave up on my dream right then. But with the encouragement of my master, I began the process of becoming a healer. It started slowly, but the pace picked up and kept growing and growing. My goal was to have people come from six countries, and now people from more than one hundred countries have come, and I've been able to help them. His Holiness The Dalai Lama came to show me his pulse many times. Mother Teresa also came to my clinic and hugged me."

"What was that like?" I wondered.

"It was like a thousand mothers hugging me. Only, when she wrapped her arms around me she asked, 'Dr. Naram, are you pregnant?' I was shocked. I didn't know what she meant until she told me she was surprised by how fat I was. At the time, I was very overweight, 220 pounds. Her question helped me see the hypocrisy of trying to bring health to others but being too busy to bring it to myself. It shocked me so much that I started studying the manuscripts to discover the ancient secrets for weight loss. I lost almost a hundred pounds."*

After that first experience of meeting Mother Teresa, Dr. Naram said she began calling him to see if he'd help people under her care. "Mother Teresa truly loved people, and so she wanted to see them heal," Dr. Naram told me. With this love, when she tried to help them with the best of modern methods that didn't work or had bad side effects, she took it personally to her heart. Then when she called Dr. Naram to help and saw people with so many problems get better, in jest, she got angry with him.

"Why did you not meet me thirty years earlier!" she said. "We could have helped so many people."

She recognized Dr. Naram had tools that helped people's ailments dissolve in a safe, nontoxic, long-term way. Dr. Naram said it was one of the happiest days of his life when Mother Teresa said, "Dr. Naram, your work is the most wonderful and purest form of healing on this planet. I really love you. Let us work together."

Bonus Material: To discover the ancient method Dr. Naram used to lose weight in a healthy way, which has helped thousands of people around the world, please refer to the videos in the free MyAncientSecrets.com membership site.

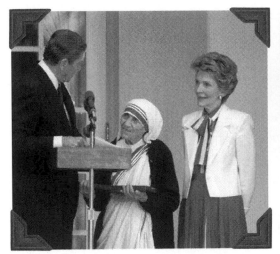
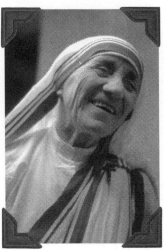

Saint Mother Teresa receiving Medal of Freedom from President Ronald Reagan in 1985. Images retrieved from Wikimedia.

Dr. Naram said, "You can love people, but if you do not have the right tools or methods to help them, then you feel frustration and pain. Especially if you try to help them with something, and how you 'help' only causes more problems. I'm so grateful my master gave me these six ancient tools, which bring deep healing. And I'm grateful Mother Teresa showed me how they are a true extension of love."

Dr. Naram then pulled out something from underneath his shirt to show me. Around his neck, under his white jacket, and hanging close to his heart were several meaningful items. There were strings of *mala* and *rudraksha* beads given to him by his master; a string of Muslim prayer pearls offered to him by a devout Muslim woman whose life Dr. Naram saved; a sacred medallion gifted by a great Sikh master; and a necklace with a Christian cross given to him by Saint Mother Teresa that had been blessed by Pope John Paul II.

"Here it is, I wanted you to see her precious gift to me. I will always treasure my time with Mother Teresa." He wrapped his fingers around the pendant with a squeeze, as if to hug it with his hand, and said, "But let's return to the point. This is about you. If you truly believe, if you truly discover what you want from your life, things can happen. Once you discover that dream or burning desire, I want to give you, over time, what my master gave to me: the tools to take that dream from your superconscious mind to your subconscious mind and to your conscious mind, to make that dream a reality in this lifetime."

I wrote this in my notes because I wanted to remember it, but also because I couldn't look him in the eyes while he was directing so much intensity and care towards me. I was insecure and riddled with uncertainty at that time in my life. I wanted to believe I could achieve clarity, but I didn't want to be disappointed if it never came.

Dr. Naram emphatically repeated, "The main point is to know what you want, achieve what you want, then enjoy what you have achieved."

I asked, "How do I do that?"

Never Chase Money; Chase Excellence

Dr. Naram said, "I'd like you to participate in a *yagna*."

A yagna is a ceremony or process with a specific objective. He said the focus of this one is discovering oneself, by asking, "Who am I? Where am I going? And how do I go further, faster, and surer, so that I am fulfilled in life?" It was no mystery why he suggested I participate.

"As a first step, I will ask Dr. Giovanni to show you what foods to eat to nourish your body and your mind, and to remain healthy, alert, focused, and full of energy, so you can achieve your dreams."

At this point, Simone found a parking spot. Before we got out of the car to walk inside the Duomo cathedral, Dr. Naram turned to me. "Clint, my master

> *"Discover for yourself: Who am I? Where am I going? And how do I go further, faster, and surer, so that I am fulfilled in life?"*
>
> –Dr. Naram

> *"Don't ever chase money. Do chase ideas, great ideas; chase and achieve great dreams."*
>
> –Baba Ramdas
> (Dr. Naram's Master)

told me something I want to tell you." With an intensity I'll never forget, he said, "Don't ever chase money. I want you to chase ideas, great ideas, and I want you to chase and achieve great dreams. Do not chase success; instead, chase and achieve excellence."

He told me that if I could discover and follow my heart's desire, the passion would come. Dr. Naram continued, "Once you are full of passion and you pursue excellence, success will come naturally. Enough money will follow, and important things in your life will occur."

"Like what?" I asked.

"You will be happy, content, and you will eventually discover fulfillment."

I quickly wrote this in my notes before we hopped out of the car. As we walked under the beautiful entrance of the cathedral, Dr. Naram said, "Only when you do this, will people truly hear you when you speak. They will notice you and you will have great impact. Believe it or not, every day everyone is influencing other people, in a positive or negative way. When you discover what you want, achieve what you want, and are enjoying what you've achieved, you become a nucleus with a ripple effect—you start in-

> *"When you discover what you want, achieve what you want, and are enjoying what you've achieved, you become a nucleus with a ripple effect—you start influencing the world in positive ways."*
>
> –Dr. Naram

fluencing the world in positive ways. And you will help make this world a healthier, happier place to live."

Dr. Naram stopped walking to look directly at me and said, "Clint, do you know why I am interested in you?"

I shook my head no, and shifted my feet. Although again in the discomfort of being the focus of attention like this, I was curious to know why he was spending so much time with me.

"It is because you are coming from

'seva.' Your actions reveal that your heart is truly about service; to your father, yes, and to everyone you meet. It just seems you are a little confused about where you can be of most service. I believe you have a role to play in helping the world become a better

> *"Going for a period of silence is one of the most insightful, powerful things you can do in life."*
>
> –Dr. Naram

place. Otherwise, why are you here? I want you to see your role, whatever it may be. I want you to know it."

My heart was beating faster with each sentence he was speaking.

"Before I found my purpose," Dr. Naram continued, "my master guided me to spend ten days in silence. This is one of the most insightful, powerful things you can do in life."

He said very few people spend so long in silence, but he did it regularly and considered it one of the most important and influential parts of his growth.

As we began walking again, he asked me, "Why do people drink? Why do people smoke? Or become addicted to food or movies or whatnot? They want to run away; they do not want to be with their inner self. They're not patient enough in their discomfort to discover the deeper layers of their being."

It became clear to me that I was stuck in the habit of running away from myself. Not with drugs or alcohol, but with work, travel, and entertainment. I saw how even my service activities were a welcome distraction from the discomfort of being with myself. I realized I didn't know who I was and didn't know how to be alone with myself long enough to find out. I had a vague idea, but it was clouded and mostly based on how I thought others saw me. To lessen my discomfort, I would work harder and play harder—or get distracted with a new relationship or with the latest electronic toy. The thrill of those moments would fizzle out quickly, and the emptiness would creep in again, telling me there must be more and I must be missing something.

As we stood outside looking up at the Duomo, Dr. Naram concluded, "There are many secrets like this. Whenever you come

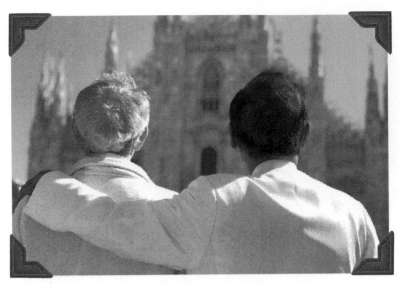

Dr. Naram with Dr. Giovanni, looking up at the Duomo.

back to India, you should go into silence. I can give you some questions to ask yourself, but first you need to enter into pure silence."

I knew this was important, but I felt frustrated by not knowing how to do more than listen. Theory is one thing, and my day-to-day reality was another. How could I take what I heard from Dr. Naram beyond the notes on my page and turn them into an actual lived experience? How could I apply them in my day-to-day life?

Your Journal Notes

To deepen and magnify the benefits you will experience from reading this book, take a few minutes now and answer the following questions for yourself.

Close your eyes, press the marmaa point on the top part of your pointer finger on your right hand, and ask yourself these questions one at a time in order. After each question, write down the first thoughts/ideas that come to you.

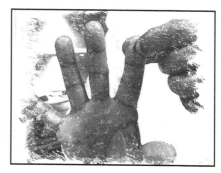

If you only had six months left to live, what would you most want to do or be?

_____

_____

_____

_____

If you knew you could not fail, what would you most want to do or be?

_____

_____

_____

_____

If you had ten million dollars in the bank and never needed to work again, what would you most want to do or be?

_____

_____

_____

_____

What other insights, questions, or realizations came to you as you read this chapter?

_____

_____

_____

_____

CHAPTER 15

Elephants, Pythons, and Priceless Moments

It is not about how much you do, but how much love you put into what you do that counts.

–Saint Mother Teresa of Calcutta

Mumbai, India

After my time in Italy, I flew to India to be with my dad. Arriving at the clinic, I was elated to see him up and walking. More than that, he glowed in a way I hadn't seen in a while. Other patients told me about the transformation they'd seen since he arrived. He smiled and said that although his body was still tender, he noticed that several of his problems were subsiding. He looked forward to going home to be retested.

During the short time I had with my father in India, Dr. Naram invited us to his home. We were greeted by his wife, Smita, who was managing all the clinics in India, including the panchakarma unit where my dad was being helped. She warmly welcomed us into her home. Upon entering, we saw Dr. Naram's ten-year-old son, Krushna, holding a humongous python.

Even in my short interactions with Krushna, I could tell he was special. Instead of being addicted to his phone or video games, like many other kids his age, Krushna was so present with us. Even though he was the son of a famous person, he was so down-to-earth humble and loving. I noticed everyone wanted to be with him, because of how good it felt to be in his presence.

"Would you like to hold it?" he asked us. Although daunting at first, it was fascinating to feel the texture, weight, and strength of the snake as its body moved through my hands, working its way up my arms to my neck as I tried to remain calm. When I said I was done, Krushna helped me untangle it from my limbs.

After we ate a delicious meal of moong soup and vegetables, someone alerted us that an elephant was out front. We fed it gourds from the garden, and as it grabbed food from our hands with its trunk, I was in awe at the sheer size of this amazing animal. At a certain point, Dr. Naram gave the elephant an instruction. With its trunk the elephant picked up a flower garland from Dr. Naram's hand and hung it around my father's neck. The smile on my dad's face was priceless.

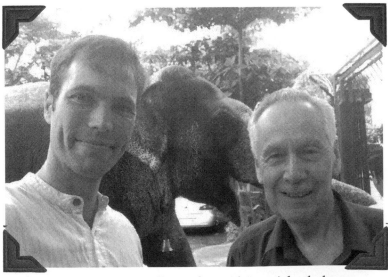

My dad and me in India together, with Laxmi the elephant.

When the elephant left, I asked Dr. Naram about the process my father was going through and the things I still worried about. I may have come across as overprotective, but it didn't stop me from inquiring about the safety and efficacy of what my father was experiencing and taking. At my impatience regarding some of the problems my dad still had, Dr. Naram said, "This is not a quick-fix program, Clint. In some situations, healing can be instantaneous. But for most cases, ancient healing works over time to heal people deeper and deeper. You can't be pregnant and tell your doctor you want to have the baby in two months, when it takes nine months. Some things just take whatever time, effort, and energy they take, whether we like it or not. My master taught me one very important thing: 'It takes time to heal yourself and others.'"

Although I understood, I was anxious to see the full results for my father. I worried about him being on such an unfamiliar path. I questioned Dr. Naram about the safety of the herbal supplements my dad was to continue taking after leaving India. Dr. Naram said, "Instead of me answering all your important questions, how about you go to the factory where they are manufactured?"

> *"This is not a quick-fix program. Ancient healing works over time to heal people deeper and deeper. My master taught me one very important thing: 'It takes time to heal yourself and others.'"*
>
> –Dr. Naram

A Fake Scientist?

Having put my father on a plane home, I spent my last couple of days in India traveling to the factories and laboratories where Dr. Naram's herbs were produced and tested. I tried to show up when they weren't expecting me.

I was immediately impressed by how clean and tidy everything was. Someone agreed to take me on a tour. I had to put covers on my shoes, sanitize my hands, and wear a hairnet. Everything was modern; the equipment for standardization and testing alone must have cost hundreds of thousands of dollars. The entire facility definitely cost millions to set up, and followed completely something that industry calls CGMP (current good manufacturing practice). Halfway through my tour, one of the administrators put me on the phone with Dr. Naram. Sincerely appreciating what I was seeing, I told him it seemed as though what he was doing was world class.

Dr. Naram quickly said, "Oh no, that's no good. My master told me we need to create the world's greatest. 'World class' is not good enough. If you see anything we can improve upon, please let me know."

He continued, "Can you imagine when I first started, I made the formulas in my own kitchen? We've come a long way. And still today, I'm ensuring, just as I did back then, that each formula we produce is made with the same love as a mother feeding her own baby."

"My master told me 'world class' is not good enough. We need to create the world's greatest."

–Dr. Naram

After my tour, I sat down and spoke with two of the scientists who had worked with Dr. Naram for decades, Dr. Pujari and Guy Kavari. Dr. Pujari proudly showed me the laboratory testing facility. "We ensure every tablet or lotion is safe, free of things like bacteria or heavy metals." He described how detailed and diligent they were to see that every bottle of herbs was standardized in terms of quality and being free of contamination. Ancient masters emphasized keeping things aligned with nature, even using the whole plant instead of extracting active ingredients. He said sometimes people are concerned because two bottles of the same herbal supplement can be different colors. He explained that because there are no artificial chemicals or dyes used, the natural variation of colors in the same plants can cause various batches of the same formula to be a slightly different hue. Just like two stocks of broccoli in a grocery market could be different shades of green, although they are both fresh broccoli. "This variation in color," he told me, "is one sign that everything is completely natural."

Dr. Pujari said that being trained in pharmaceutical research, he hadn't believed in the ancient healing science at all. Then he did his own testing and the results proved the effectiveness of these herbs and methods.

Guy Kavari explained that soon after he started working with Dr. Naram, it was evident there was no existing codex or database in India, in Ayurveda, or anywhere in the West for the herbs and procedures Dr. Naram was interested in using. They built a new laboratory, painstakingly testing hundreds of herbs, documenting their properties, and creating their own library of them.

When I asked Guy how he'd describe Dr. Naram as a person, without hesitation he said, "Two words: humanitarian and genius."

It surprised me that he said this so quickly and confidently. "Why?" I asked.

He said most people in this industry just wanted to cut costs, so they got the cheapest raw products and fastest processing methods. Dr. Naram, on the other hand, wanted the highest quality regardless of the price or time it took.

"Is that why his herbs are more expensive than most other herbal supplements?" I asked.

Guy said he knew the cost of producing the herbal products this way, and also the price for which Dr. Naram was selling them. "There is barely any profit for him. For that passion, I call him a humanitarian."

"And why genius?" I asked.

"Years ago, before the governments of India or America were even concerned about heavy metals, Dr. Naram insisted that any products he created would have to be heavy-metal free. So from the very beginning, they found the best raw materials and innovative processes to ensure each product was free of heavy metals, regardless of the cost or effort it took."

Later, I told Dr. Naram my experience at the factory. He told me how grateful he was for the people I met. They made certain the

ancient processes were followed. They also guaranteed that each formula passed the highest standards of modern nutraceutical testing.

Dr. Naram confided in me about problems, disagreements,
and difficulties he often had when working with a new scientist.
The processes his master and the ancient texts encouraged were
vastly different from what was taught or understood in today's
universities. Scientists didn't understand Dr. Naram's insistence in
making sure certain mantras were spoken before and during the
production of the herbs, or why things were to be combined only
in certain ways and at certain times. Especially when it took longer
and cost more than doing it a simpler way.

In the case of Guy Kavari, the conflict came when Dr. Naram
said that a certain herb that eased heavy bleeding during women's
menstrual period needed to be harvested only at midnight on a
full moon. Guy thought this was nonsense and told Dr. Naram so.
He said that as a scientist he wouldn't believe in fairy tales and
refused to harvest that herb at midnight.

"You are actually not a scientist at all," Dr. Naram responded
"You are fake."

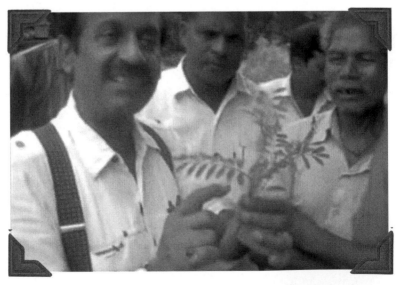

*Dr. Naram in rural area where herbs are collected, holding a plant
which has juice that helps reduce pain and boost immunity.*

Guy was caught off guard and defended himself. "I am a scientist; that is why I don't believe this nonsense."

"You are a fake scientist, believing something to be true that you don't know," Dr. Naram said. "If you were a true scientist, you'd know you have a hypothesis, but not a conclusion. And you would test it, to see what is true."

Guy felt as if he was tossed a challenge he couldn't decline, so he designed an extensive study to prove Dr. Naram wrong. He harvested that specific herb at different times of the day, including at midnight on a full moon. Then he tested the potency of the active ingredient with their equipment. He took the various samples, mixed them into the formula, and gave them to women who had the bleeding problem.

The results were shocking to Guy. The potency of the herbs harvested at midnight on a full moon was almost twenty times higher than the exact same herb when harvested during the day. When mixed into the supplement and given to women who needed it, the results were clearly better. From that point onward, Guy agreed to follow the procedure of harvesting the herbs and mixing the formulas exactly as was outlined in the ancient healing manuscripts.

He discovered other fascinating results in their laboratory, which ran contrary to his training. To his surprise, the rancidity levels decreased and shelf life increased when following specifications in the ancient texts.

My questions about the safety of the herbs were resolved. At the same time, I was inspired to see people working with so much passion and excellence.

Disturbing Email from My Dad

From India, I flew through Thailand to China, to give a presentation at an academic conference. I was surrounded by professors and students talking about the various developments in technology and how they would affect education. After spending time with Dr. Naram, going back to my "normal" life was disorienting, to say the least.

The way I saw myself and the world was changing. When I tried to share with others some of the things I'd witnessed, they often gave me a look of disbelief that would end the conversation. I decided it wasn't my role to convince anyone of anything. My dad was better and that was all that mattered to me.

When I arrived in China, I emailed my mom and dad to let them know I was safe, and asked how they were doing. Within a day, I received troubling news from my father.

September 10, 2010

Hi Son,

You constantly amaze me. You talk about staying the night in Bangkok and going to China before traveling to the next country as if you spent the night in Provo and were on your way to our house in Salt Lake City.

I am still trying to recover from my trip to India. After getting home I experienced an energy meltdown. Not able to do much of anything. Thanks for giving us your schedule. When will you next connect with Dr. Naram? If soon, I have a couple of questions you may be able to get answers for, as I don't understand what is happening in my body.

Please know you are in my prayers that your trip will be safe and fruitful for everyone involved.

Love you lots,
Dad

I quickly wrote him back with the contact information for Dr. Naram's call center, which would connect him. I felt the uneasy, quiet sadness coming back to enfold me again. After all this time, expense, and effort, had ancient healing and Dr. Naram failed my dad?

Your Journal Notes

To deepen and magnify the benefits you will experience from reading this book, take a few minutes now and answer the following questions for yourself:

Name one or two things, that if you did them in your life with even more excellence, would change everything:

_____

_____

_____

_____

What good things in your life have come as a result of patience and discipline?

_____

_____

_____

_____

What other insights, questions, or realizations came to you as you read this chapter?

_____

_____

_____

_____

CHAPTER 16

An Unexpected New Problem

Don't say, 'It is morning,' and dismiss it with a name of yesterday.
See it for the first time as a newborn child that has no name.

–Rabindranath Tagore

After China, I returned to Finland to my work at the University of Joensuu (which later became the University of Eastern Finland). I was living in a small town, covered in snow, not far from the Russian border. Although I have a deep love of Finland, the people, and my work there, after his disturbing email I felt a pressing need to see my dad. This feeling grew when my dad called to ask when I'd be home again to discuss his health in person. He mentioned "a new problem." I was anxious and confused and flew home as soon as I could.

Standing outside the door of my parents' home, I wondered what my dad wanted to discuss. It had been over six months since I first introduced him to Dr. Naram in LA. Was he any better? Would I notice a change in him? Or did I send him halfway around the world for nothing? Was he still suffering? Was he getting worse? Only half a year prior, he told me he might not live to see the next morning. The memory was still fresh and tender.

My dad greeted me at the door with a look I couldn't read. We walked into his office and sat in the same chairs we sat in the last time I was there. Only this time, instead of looking at the ground, he didn't break eye contact with me.

Settling in, he took a deep breath. "Son, there's a new problem."

My heart sank. Bracing myself, I asked, "What do you mean?"

From behind his desk he pulled out a shoebox and opened it. It was filled with bottles of pills. "My problem is I don't know what to do with all these pills. I don't need them anymore!" A huge smile swept across his face. Out of the twelve medications he'd been taking before India, he now only needed one. I stopped holding my breath and let out a big sigh of relief! His smile was contagious and I laughed with surprise.

It turned out that the energy meltdown he experienced after India was momentary, occurring because he started eating all the familiar old food he wasn't supposed to eat. So he suffered the consequences. Once he took the home remedies and adjusted his diet again, he immediately started feeling better.

I couldn't believe it. Only half a year earlier, he was in excruciating pain and didn't know how much longer he'd live. His body was so weak, even simple things like getting up out of a chair or walking down the hallway were monumental challenges. He was consumed by a weariness that terrified me. With his mind slipping toward Alzheimer's, he'd lose track of a sentence and readily forget things. And it was heartbreaking to watch him slide into severe depression.

Now, only a few months after meeting Dr. Naram and being disciplined in following his advice, my dad was a changed man. He no longer had cholesterol problems, his blood pressure was normal, and he didn't struggle with blood sugar problems anymore. During the process, he had periodic meetings with his regular doctors, who monitored his progress and were surprised to soon be recommending he didn't need certain medications anymore. By the time I met him, he was almost completely free of needing any!

Perhaps most significant for my dad was that all the pain in his legs and chest was gone, so now he was off painkillers, too. "In fact," he said, "there's no pain in my entire body!"

He described how he had twenty times more energy, physical ability and mental alertness. He could work again and feel as though he was making a difference on the planet. Watching my dad feeling useful and productive, contributing to the greater good, as was always his mission, made me feel more fulfilled than ever before.

My mind was racing. Could this really be happening?

What a holy moment! What a beautiful gift!

Even as I write this, reflecting back on that moment, tears flow down my cheeks in gratitude.

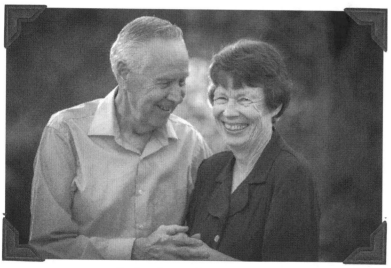

Dad and Mom laughing again.

The most meaningful moment was when my dad looked me squarely in the eye and said, "Now I have another important request for you, Son."

Taking their rightful place on top of my dad's desk, instead of shoved back into the drawer, was the stack of folders and papers with all the materials he had collected over his lifetime. Remember that book he wanted to write, synthesizing his life's work of helping children recognize good ideas and make good choices? When he was ill and depression consumed him, my dad lost sight and hope of that goal.

Placing his hand atop the stack of papers, he said, "I want to finish writing *The Missing Piece in Education,* and I want your help. Son, will you be my coauthor?"

I was beyond honored, and even though I couldn't stop smiling, tears were pouring down my face.

"Absolutely," I told him.

What a different request from the one he made six months earlier! I hoped writing this book would be healing for my dad, something gratifying that would become part of his legacy. Little did I know it would heal me, too. But that is a story for another time.

After my dad's remarkable recovery, I started describing what Dr. Naram did for people as an oil change for your body. When you change the filters in your car, you can see how much gunk has accumulated. We don't see it in our bodies, but it's there. If we don't cleanse it and take proper care, it manifests as a malfunction. When the filters in my dad's body were cleaned, his health problems cleared up.

Feeling grateful for Dr. Naram and this ancient healing system, and seeing with my own eyes the amazing transformation my father experienced, I called Dr. Naram to thank him, but there was no answer. What I didn't know was that, as my father's health steadily improved, Dr. Naram's father slipped into a coma and was declared dead.

Your Journal Notes

To deepen and magnify the benefits you will experience from reading this book, take a few minutes now and answer the following questions for yourself:

Who is someone you love? Do you know their biggest dream?

_____

_____

_____

_____

_____

How can you support them in achieving it? Or how can you help them become more clear, if they're not yet sure what they want?

_____

_____

_____

_____

_____

What other insights, questions, or realizations came to you as you read this chapter?

_____

_____

_____

_____

CHAPTER 17

Saying Goodbye

What is the most remarkable thing in all the world?
That everyone will die, but no one ever
thinks it will happen to them.

–Paraphrased from the Bhagavad Gita, a 5,000-year-old text

D r. Naram knew his father was not well. He visited him many
times in the last years and was always able to help him. This
time, his father's prognosis was dire. Before heading to his parents'
home, Dr. Naram invited Dr. Giovanni, Luciano, and Vinay with
him, unsure of what he would face.

When they arrived, they were tearfully greeted at the entrance
by Dr. Naram's brother, Vidyutt, his mother, the rest of his family,
and the doctor, who was just completing the death certificate. It
was too late.

"I want to see him." Dr. Naram told his brother.

Dr. Naram walked up next to the bed where his father's body
was resting. He reached out to hold his father's wrist and was startled to notice something. His fingers detected a very faint pulse. He
immediately asked Dr. Giovanni to get the blood pressure machine
and test his blood pressure and pulse. Dr. Giovanni did and the

machine showed there was no pulse. Dr. Naram asked him to test again, and same result, no pulse, no blood pressure.

Dr. Naram asked Dr. Giovanni to quickly get ginger and ajwain powder from the kitchen. Everyone in the house asked Dr. Giovanni why he needed them. The attending doctor also looked up with a puzzled expression on his face, and the family explained to him that Dr. Naram was a pulse healer. He shook his head and went back to his paperwork.

Dr. Naram instructed Dr. Giovanni to rub the dry mixture of ajwain and ginger powders on his father's feet. Simultaneously, Dr. Naram put ghee on and pressed specific marmaa points on his hands, feet, belly, and head. After several minutes, he leaned close to his father's ear and said, "Papa, if you are aware, if you can hear me and want to live, then raise your hand, your feet, or even your finger. If not, they are going to take your body to burn you now."

His father lifted his whole hand!

Dr. Naram couldn't contain his excitement, telling his brother that their father was still alive. The attending doctor was skeptical and accused Dr. Naram of moving his father's hand himself. Everyone came into the room and watched as Dr. Naram repeated the procedure. This time, his father lifted his entire leg up, and the attending doctor jumped back in shock.

As I listened to this part, I laughed, imagining the whole scene. The doctor thought it might be rigor mortis until Dr. Naram continued the process. Dr. Naram's father loved the guru Sai Baba. Knowing this, Dr. Naram asked Dr. Giovanni to help press the marmaa points and while doing so speak the common greeting of Sai Baba devotees, "Sai Ram." A faint yet clear reply came from the bed, "Sai Ram."

Everyone was stunned. Through a huge smile of amazement, Dr. Giovanni said again, "Sai Ram."

An ever louder "Sai Ram!" came from Dr. Naram's father. Upon hearing this, everyone in the room laughed with joy, several of them through tears.

Only the doctor was not smiling. With the signed death certificate still wet with ink, this was beyond his comprehension. He declared this man dead, and now he was speaking? Instead of saying goodbye to their father that night, the family said goodbye to the doctor. He was speechless as he walked out the door.

"It is important that we complete certain things in life so our souls can rest in peace."
–Dr. Naram

Dr. Naram's father, awake and aware, recovered enough over the next week that he could sit up, walk, and speak with his family. The attending doctor who signed the death certificate called Dr. Naram's brother every few days for an update on "that strange case." Each time, he was surprised to learn that the patient was still alive and thriving.

Dr. Naram's father soon felt well enough to complete some unfinished business, sign important documents, and have vital conversations with his wife, children, and grandchildren.

"It is important that we complete certain things in life so our souls can rest in peace," Dr. Naram shared.

When I expressed how remarkable that was, Dr. Naram repeated the words of his master: "Never give up hope!"

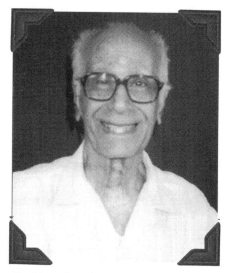

Dr. Naram's Father, Khimjibhai U Naram.

My Journal Notes

Additional Ancient Healing Secrets for Helping Someone in a Coma* (Continued from Chapter 1)

4) Home Remedy—Mix dry ginger powder and ajwain powder together and rub on the feet of the person in a coma.

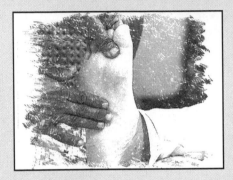

5) Marmaa Shakti—While pressing the points outlined in chapter 1 (on page 15), speak the person's name in a way that is most familiar to them.

*Bonus Material: To hear Dr. Giovanni & Dr. Naram talk about this moment, and for you to understand this method more deeply, please refer to the free MyAncientSecrets.com membership site.

Your Journal Notes

To deepen and magnify the benefits you will experience from reading this book, take a few minutes now and answer the following questions for yourself:

What things in your life would you love to complete before you die (e.g., face some fear, forgive someone, achieve something, ask forgiveness from someone, overcome some challenge, etc.)?

_____

_____

_____

_____

_____

What other insights, questions, or realizations came to you as you read this chapter?

_____

_____

_____

_____

_____

CHAPTER 18

Ancient Wisdom, Modern World

All journeys have secret destinations
of which the traveler is unaware.

−Martin Buber

Soon after these seemingly miraculous events, Dr. Naram invited me to an awards ceremony in New Jersey, where he was being honored for helping 9/11 firefighters and first responders. As I stood among thousands of people talking and waiting for the ceremony to start, I knew in my heart I needed to ask Dr. Naram a question that had been nagging me for a while.

I smiled when I spotted Marshall and José, two of the founders of *Serving Those Who Serve*, whom I had met earlier in New York. They were now helping people who survived other disasters and hoped Dr. Naram would continue to support them.

Dr. Naram smiled when he saw me. "So glad you could come, Clint."

I was honored to be there. "Are you excited?" I asked. "I heard the Governor of New Jersey is here to give you the award."

"More like humbled," he replied.

"Why is that?"

"I know power is in this lineage, the secrets recorded in the ancient texts and the teachings of my master. I am simply a translator of this ancient wisdom for the modern world. And speaking of my master, do you know the story of how I knew what could help these firefighters of 9/11?"

"How?"

"Street kids in Mumbai!" he said.

"Street kids?"

"Yes, after the thousand days of training, my master gave me a service, or *seva* (pronounced *say-vah*) assignment. He told me that the first people I was assigned to help were in Dharavi, the second largest slum in the world."

Dr. Naram described how he met the street kids living there, with their dirty faces and torn clothes. He felt their pulse and gave them herbs he thought would help them. But when he went back, he discovered none worked and the kids were still sick with lung problems, sleeping issues, depression, anxiety, and coughing, and their pulse still showed a buildup of toxins in their bodies. Confused, Dr. Naram consulted with his master and was told he needed to go deeper and learn more about these children.

Dr. Naram went back and asked the kids where they lived and worked. He found out they worked in a chemical factory. The factory didn't want to pay for machines to stir the tubs of chemicals, so hired the street kids to swim around in them. He was shocked, reported this to the authorities, and went back to his master to find out what else he could do to help these children.

Together, they studied the manuscripts to see if anything was used in ancient times to help remove difficult toxins, like heavy metals. They got excited when they discovered a possible solution. In ancient wars, soldiers dipped the tips of their arrows and spears in chemical poisons. The healers in the Siddha-Veda lineage needed to find ways to help people release the poison. They identified twenty-seven herbs (including turmeric and neem) that could help remove these toxic heavy metals. Based on what they found, Dr. Naram and his master created a new formula, in order to try it with the street kids.

"It worked, and the children got better! The toxins were eradicated from their bodies. My faith in the principles from my

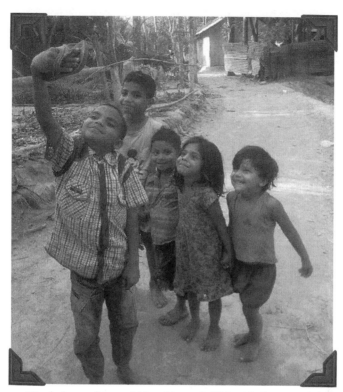

Viral photo of street kids taking a 'selfie' with their sandal.
Retrieved from Google Images.

master and these ancient texts increased, seeing them help in such a dramatic case. Then 9/11 happened, and it was something the world and America had never seen."

When Dr. Naram was invited to help the firefighters who worked day and night in the pit at Ground Zero, he knew they, too, had similar toxins in their bodies from inhaling fumes and being in contact with so much toxic debris. He also knew that Western medicine did not yet have a way to remove these toxins. "It was my pleasure and honor to be of service. I thank my master for teaching me how to be so useful to people in need. Everyone, even in daily life, is polluted to some degree as well. Everyone inhales exhaust fumes from cars and trucks, eats processed or modified foods which are often watered by acid rain, is exposed to cell phone radiation, eats meat or plants that are polluted, and experiences a different quality of sunlight because of atmosphere issues with the ozone layer. So even if we weren't in New York on 9/11, we all need these ancient secrets to remove environmental toxins from our bodies."

Though it was all very fascinating, I could not forget the burning question I needed to ask him. Just as I was about to open my mouth, someone interrupted us to take Dr. Naram to the stage.

I sat in my chair in the audience, and I read the program containing more stories from the firefighters and first responders who benefited from Dr. Naram's help. One of them was Darren Taylor, an FDNY firefighter. He wrote:

"I was dispatched to Ground Zero two days after the World Trade Center attacks. I was working in general body recovery and search, and for general reconnaissance and fire suppression. I started noticing effects to my health about a month after working regular tours in the city. I was getting colds more frequently. Sometimes I woke up at night with a coughing fit, a nonproductive dry cough. I was a bit depressed, and my immune system was impacted negatively. I was feeling sicker in general—not as healthy as I normally was. When I first heard about this program and these herbs, I wasn't interested. But months after I was at Ground Zero, my symptoms got worse. I was concerned about them and figured I would try something natural. I'm glad I did. After taking the herbs for a while, I found that my colds were pretty much taken care of and my coughing fits faded away. I had

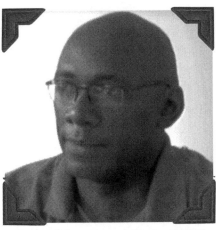

9/11 Firefighter Darren Taylor, FDNY, used Dr. Naram's herbs to remove toxins from his body, boost immunity, improve sleep, and live a much healthier and happier life!

more stamina. I just felt better. I was less depressed. I was more able to go on with my life and put the medical concerns behind me. I got more sleep, and better sleep. Now, I feel really well in general. Thanks to all of you for the service you offer. Good luck with getting it to more people."

Another first responder said she'd been taking the herbs for about a year when something amazing happened: her pulmonary function tests showed normal readings and, for the first time in years, she could go off her inhalers. She wrote:

"And there's a side benefit; I was able to stop smoking entirely with the herbs. I could smell the cigarettes coming out of my body. Even though I quit smoking for a year, I always had a craving. Then whatever storage of nicotine was in the pockets of my body, I think the herbs got rid of them. Sometimes I would urinate and it would smell like an ashtray. I'd be like, 'Where did that come from?' And I think that the herbs released the nicotine out of my system. Everything has improved so much in the course of the last year, and I attribute it to Dr. Naram's herbs. I guess they take poison out of every part of your body."

I carried on reading story after story like this. I thought about how powerful it was that José was guided to meet Dr. Naram and set up this organization to help the 9/11 first responders. I bet he had no idea when he first met Dr. Naram that this was the path his life would take.

Then I thought back to Reshma and Rabbat. She probably had no clue when she first watched Dr. Naram on television that she'd be guided to meet him to save her daughter's life. When Dr. Giovanni first met Dr. Naram, he didn't have a clue that his whole life would be devoted to learning the ancient healing secrets and utilizing them with his patients. My mind was directed to the unexpected guidance and miracle of it all.

Just then, I remembered a prayer I had said when I was a child, struggling with my sister Denise's death. I prayed that God would guide me to wherever I could be of most service, so I could help those who were in pain.

I closed my eyes and my mind opened up to the mystery of what had unfolded since then. My sister's death led me to Gary Malkin and the Wisdom of the World project. To help it succeed, I met Gail Kingsbury, and she introduced me to Dr. Naram. My crush on Alicia led me to India. My dad's declining health led me to investigate the ancient healing secrets more deeply, and so on. In each case, I was amazed to see that the best things in my life happened when I was trying to be of service to others. It was clear that at those times, especially when my heart was focused on helping others, a higher divine power led me to where healing was provided for us all. A little overwhelmed by the flood of realizations, I wondered where life would lead me now.

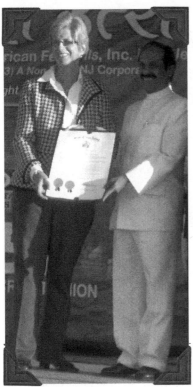

Dr. Naram receiving an award from the State of New Jersey, given by the Honorable Former Governor Christine Todd Whitman, for helping thousands of 9/11 Firefighters & First Responders.

When I heard the announcer speak into the microphone, I opened my eyes and focused my attention on the stage. After general introductions and formalities, the now former governor of New Jersey, Christine Todd Whitman, came to the microphone. She thanked Dr. Naram for helping thousands of 9/11 firefighters, police officers, and other first responders. She held up the award being given by the state legislature of New Jersey to Dr. Naram, and read a section of what it said: "The Senate and General Assembly of the State of New Jersey are pleased to salute and proudly honor Dr. Pankaj Naram, a highly esteemed specialist of ancient healing and pulse diagnosis, renowned for his philanthropic efforts, for exemplifying the spirit of caring and compassion in service to the first responders of the terrorist attack of 9/11, for his distinguished record of service to our community in the health field, and for promoting his ancient healing science throughout the world."

Governor Whitman finished reading the letter, then asked Dr. Naram to come to the stage. She proudly shook his hand and presented him with the award. She guided him to the microphone, his white suit contrasting with the dark colors behind him. Dr. Naram began to speak in his own special way.

"Namaste. I am being given this award to be honored along with the founders of *Serving Those Who Serve*—Marshall, José, Nechemiah, and Rosemary. But the real heroes of the day are the firefighters, police, and others who went to the heart of the danger and risked their lives. The least we can do is help them get their health and their lives back.

"In my lineage of healers, we do not consider ourselves heroes. We see those who come to us as doing us a favor by allowing us to use our ancient methods to help them. My master said this was one way to enlightenment. What do people do in order to achieve happiness, or what we call *moksha*, which is enlightenment, or fulfillment? Some take the path of meditation, some the path of prayer, some success in business or in battle. In India, we call these paths *karmayog*, *bhaktiyog*, or *gyanyog*. According to my master, on the path of a healer you get enlightenment or fulfillment only if your patients are happy. Helping people heal is our source for enlightenment and happiness. We treat each person as a temple. You can say a patient is a temple or a church, or a mosque, or a *gurudwara*. These are all names of places of worship. My master taught me that God resides in each of us, so you are a temple. Now if this is true, then when does God become happy? When you clean the temple! Each person has many compartments like mind, emotions, and soul. When these are cleaned, we experience a transformation physically, mentally, and emotionally. As a result, we can go on to achieve whatever we want to in life. I'm so grateful to my master for teaching me the principles of the ancient science which brings these deeper transformative possibilities to anyone who uses it."

As he spoke, I thought of the smile on my father's face when he showed me the box of medications he no longer needed. I was so grateful Dr. Naram helped to flush the toxins from his body, rebalancing his doshas. I smiled that I even knew what that word *dosha* meant now! I wondered what other ancient principles I could learn that would help me and others. I thought about the eleven-year-old girl Rabbat coming out of her coma, saying "Mommy" when she awoke, and the tears in her mother's eyes. I reflected on the nurse's jubilation that the same method helped her own sister too. I thought of Rabbi Stephen Robbins from California, going from his deathbed and needing a wheelchair to now working out in the gym again, looking and feeling ten years younger. I remembered the man with the frozen shoulder getting full mobility, Giovanni and the bee-keepers rescuing their hive, the woman having a baby after menopause, and so many of the people who told me "Dr. Naram saved my life." I reflected on the people at Dr. Naram's factory making the herbs according to the ancient ways, with so much precision and love, and all the firefighters who benefited from them.

"This is known as *seva*, or service, of a healer. My master taught me it is seva not for the patient, but for the healer," Dr. Naram continued. "My master also taught me the healer needs to take care of two obstacles first, in order to help people. Which are the two obstacles? Ego and fear.

"In the midst of unspeakable danger, these great firefighters, police officers, and others who helped on 9/11 left behind ego and fear. They are great examples of the kind of true seva, or service, that brings fulfillment. My master taught me God is here in each of you. And it is my honor to serve the divine hero in each of you, in whatever way I can."

The audience erupted in a standing ovation. As Dr. Naram came down from the stage, a crowd of people surrounded him. Watching him, I felt my heart swelling with full appreciation for who he is, what he dedicates his life to, and how it has blessed so many people.

As I went from watching Dr. Naram to looking inward again,

I saw that the skeptic I originally was had almost totally melted away. Beyond that, I felt a sense of purpose and a deeper peace than I ever felt before in my life. It wasn't a journey I had planned to take, but nonetheless life had brought me on this path, and I felt it must be for a reason. Sure, there were still a lot of grey areas—so many things I could not make sense of yet. But instead of automatically discounting those things, my mind opened into to a relentless curiosity about them, desiring to test them out for myself and discover how they worked.

It was only later that evening that Dr. Naram and I had a moment together again, when I could finally ask my burning question.

The Burning Question

With the crowds finally gone, there was a moment of quiet when only Dr. Naram and I were waiting for the car that would soon come get him. He spoke of his master and told me how proud he imagined his beloved Baba Ramdas would be to see the ancient secrets helping people all over the world in the deepest of ways. "Do you know one of the greatest secrets for happiness and success, Clint? Gratitude. Always give credit to those who have taught you."

Speaking from a most tender place, Dr. Naram shared, "Before my master left his body, he helped me discover my life's work and mission. He taught me that this mission is beyond nation, beyond religion, beyond politics, beyond caste, creed, and race. It is for *all* humanity. He said that ancient healing is like a lotus flower. Do you know about the lotus flower?"

Dr. Naram's sister Varsha once told me that Dr. Naram's first name, Pankaj, when translated into English means "lotus."

> *"One of the greatest secrets for happiness and success is—gratitude. Always give credit to those who have taught you."*
>
> –Dr. Naram

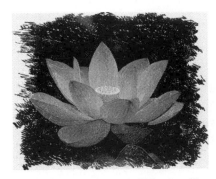

Dr. Naram's master said he should be like a lotus flower.

"My master said just as the brilliant white lotus flower rises out of the dark mud to share its brightness and fragrance with us all, so must these ancient healing secrets open up to reveal their deeper healing beauty and power with all humanity. It is not a religion, a cult, or anything like that. It is simply a school of thought that anyone can join and benefit from—by learning how to help themselves and others to heal deeper and deeper. My master also helped me discover my mission—to protect, preserve, and bring the benefits of these secrets into every heart and every home on earth."

I listened, impressed by the state of gratitude from which Dr. Naram spoke. Not able to wait any longer, I said, "Dr. Naram, can I ask you an important question?"

He nodded.

"I'm convinced that more people need to know that these ancient healing techniques are an option. What you know and do can help so many people on this planet. They may not choose to do it, but at least they should know it's a choice." Finally, my burning question jumped out of my mouth, "How can I help you?"

The palpably serious moment shifted as Dr. Naram cracked a smile and let out a quiet but audible laugh in response to my question. I was so confused, it must have shown on my face. He said, "Thank you, Clint. I want help and need help. Only, not from you."

> *"This mission of ancient healing is beyond nation, beyond religion, beyond politics, beyond caste, creed, and race. It is for all humanity. It is a school of thought, that anyone can benefit from—by learning how to help themselves and others to heal deeper and deeper."*
>
> –Dr. Naram

I was shocked. My brow furrowed as I tried to figure out whether I'd heard him correctly.

He said, "I know you now, and your mind is way too crowded." He laughed again.

"I . . . I don't understand."

Dr. Naram looked at me kindly and said, "You now know Siddha-Veda's six keys of deeper healing. Hopefully, you will get to know each of them more by using them to benefit your life and the lives of others. But right now, Clint, even if I shared with you some of the other most basic secrets that my master taught me, you would not understand them properly. You'd try to figure them out with your intellect, not understand them with your heart or integrate them into your being. Like I said, your mind is way too crowded."

At a loss, I asked, "What can I do, then?"

"I'm willing to share with you so many things, even deeper secrets, once you are ready." He paused, then continued, "But before you can really help me, there is something you need to do for yourself first."

"I want to learn. I'll do anything! What do you want me to do?"

Dr. Naram smiled and said, "Come tomorrow."

Your Journal Notes

To deepen and magnify the benefits you will experience from reading this book, take a few minutes now and answer the following questions for yourself:

What are you most grateful for in your life?

_____

_____

_____

_____

Whom have you felt guided to meet in your life, that you could contact today and express gratitude toward?

_____

_____

_____

_____

What other insights, questions, or realizations came to you as you read this chapter and completed this book?

_____

_____

_____

_____

Dedication

I dedicate this book in special memory of my sister
Denise.
I love you always.

I may not have had the tools or knowledge to help you while you
were alive ... but I dedicate this book in your name, hoping it
leads many people to find hope and a path of deeper healing.

And special dedication to legendary master healer,
Dr. Naram.

Thank you for devoting your life force to mastering and
sharing these ancient healing secrets, for the benefit
of every home and every heart on earth.

Dear Reader,

Thank you for reading this, Book #1, and joining along with me during the first year of my life-changing journey with Dr. Naram!

In the remaining pages, I've put an Afterword (with an update on what's happened since then, and how it applies to you), an Author's Note (with info on a priceless gift I have for you), and an appendix (with a glossary of new words, some bonus ancient secret remedies, and other helpful information, too).

First, however, I wanted to share a short epilogue I think you will enjoy.

Divine Guidance, Self-Healing Secrets, and the Principles for Manifesting Your Dreams into Reality

Don't write your name on the sand, waves will wash it away.
Don't write your name in the sky, wind may blow it away.
Write your name in the hearts of people you come in touch with.
That's where it will stay.

–Author Unknown

Dhaka, Bangladesh (Three years later)

The plane landed. Dr. Giovanni and I entered the airport, not sure what to expect. Though we often traveled together during the four years since we first met, neither of us had been to Bangladesh. Our trepidation quickly dissipated. The immigration officers and border guards were friendly, helpful, and funny. I found out that Bangladesh separated from India as part of Pakistan in 1947, before it emerged as an independent nation in 1971. Since then, the country has had two female prime ministers. I had to face my own prejudice about what a Muslim country would be like. Whereas

American media emphasized how some Islamic states wouldn't let women drive a car, I was surprised this Islamic country already had their second female prime minister. In the United States, we've not yet had one female president.

After retrieving our bags, we met Kalim Hussain in the lobby.

"*As-salaam Walaykum*," he said to us, the traditional greeting in Bangladesh, meaning "Peace be unto you."

Before arriving, I learned the proper response: "*Walaykum—as salaam,*" meaning, "And unto you."

"My daughter is very much looking forward to seeing you," he said.

We walked outside the airport and saw several people, including a beautiful young woman. As we got closer, I recognized her eyes—and her smile. I stared in awe.

"As-salaam Walaykum, Dr. Clint, Dr. Giovanni," she said.

Rabbat was now fourteen. I wondered, *Who was this person, so beautiful, so intelligent, so alive?* She was none other than the little girl who came out of the coma in the Mumbai hospital. Though her appearance had transformed entirely in the three years since we saw her, her voice was exactly the same. Its gentle and rhythmic intonation was soothing to my ears and soul.

"*Walaykum—as salaam,*" I said, barely able to speak.

I couldn't keep my eyes off her. Her English was even better than when we met, and she exuded incredible kindness and confidence. I didn't wait long before asking if I could take a picture. As she stood next to Dr. Giovanni, I noticed they were almost the same height now.

A year earlier, I received a Facebook friend request but didn't recognize who it was from at first. I was delighted to realize it was Rabbat! It brought back all the emotions of her amazing recovery. *How interesting this world is*, I thought. *How intricately interconnected we all are.*

Once we got in the car, I asked her something I had been wondering: "Why is your Facebook name *Swan Bella*?"

"You know the book *Twilight*?" she asked.

"Yes."

"That is the main character's name."

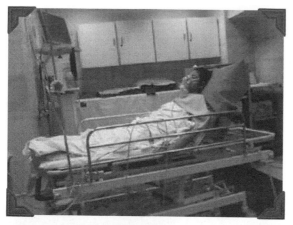

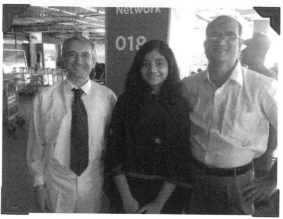

Top: Rabbat when we first met her in the hospital in Mumbai.
Bottom: With Dr. Giovanni and her father at the airport in Dhaka.

"Have you read the book?" I asked.

"No, I just liked the name."

We both laughed.

"How are you doing now?" I asked her.

"Strong as a horse."

Once we arrived at her home, Rabbat's mother, Reshma, her brother, and several relatives greeted us. Reshma was overjoyed to welcome us.

"In Bangladesh we have a tradition to give something sweet to our guests," she said, bringing out a plate filled with a variety of sweets I'd never seen before.

"We also have a gift for you," Dr. Giovanni said.

"No, the gift is yourself, that you came. We are so happy," Reshma said.

Dr. Giovanni brought out several bracelets and medallions for Rabbat and her family, from Dr. Naram.

They fed us a fantastic meal with rice and vegetables followed by even more sweets. We talked, sometimes struggling to understand each other, but laughing and smiling a lot.

After the meal, Rabbat and Daanish (pronounced *Dah-nish*), one of her two younger brothers, walked with us to see their school.

Daanish had the same dark hair, sparkly eyes, and curiosity about the world that Rabbat did. Easygoing, friendly, and clearly very intelligent, he had a contagious enthusiasm about life.

As the four of us walked the narrow street to the school, we passed food vendors and shops where people lingered in the doorways. Cows and chickens roamed the streets, and we stopped to feed them. Rabbat and Daanish bought coconuts from a cart, one for each of us, and the vendor used his sharp knife to crack them open. We drank the sweet water straight from the shell, and Daanish showed me how to eat the white pulp inside.

A couple of little girls were following us, and I thought they might be hungry, so I offered them some of my coconut. They turned around and ran away as fast as they could, disappearing behind a corner. A moment later, we saw them peaking around it, looking at us, talking and giggling to each other. I soon noticed everyone we passed on the streets was looking at us.

"They are curious," said Daanish, laughing. "They don't often see foreigners like you."

"How can they tell we are foreigners?" I asked.

"You are so tall, and your skin is so pale. You know what we call people like you?"

"What?"

"Dead people," he said. "Because your skin is so pale it looks like you are already dead. You look like a vampire."

We laughed at how funny that sounded.

By the time we got to the school, we had a large group of kids following us. Wanting to connect with them, I asked, through Daanish, if they would sing a song. They started singing the national anthem of Bangladesh, their young voices joining together harmoniously.

More kids and a few adults gathered to see what was happening. As soon as they finished their song, Dr. Giovanni got up in front of everyone and sang the national anthem of Italy. Everyone loved it.

I couldn't wait to call home and tell my mom and dad about the amazing and profound experience of seeing Rabbat and being in Bangladesh. I knew my dad thoroughly loved hearing each fun and fascinating detail of my travels.

As Rabbat showed us the school, she explained it was an English language school, and that one of her best subjects was math. She gave us an example: "When I was in a coma, the head doctor at the hospital recommended taking me off life support and letting me die. Another doctor gave me a 10 percent chance of survival. But Dr. Naram took that 10 percent and squared it."

"What do you mean?" Dr. Giovanni asked.

"He squared it." She explained, "Ten squared equals ten times ten. Dr. Naram gave me 100 percent chance of survival."

We all smiled and laughed.

"How do you feel now?" I asked.

"Now I feel 110 percent."

Then, Rabbat became serious. "Mother told me she gave up everything," she said. "When she took me to India for my treatments at the hospital, all our money was spent. She was separated from my father, her other children, our family, home—everything. We lost a lot, and yet she said she found and won the thing that mattered most—my life."

Rabbat and Daanish took us to meet other family members living nearby. Everyone gave us sweets, and Dr. Giovanni and I, already full, politely took the smallest ones. We met the parents of one of their younger cousins who, we learned, was ill and vomiting.

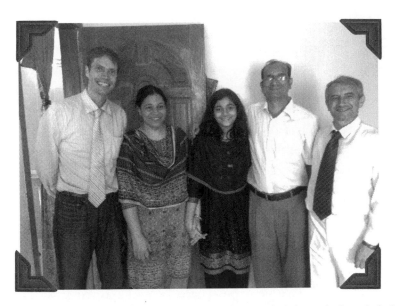

Me, Reshma, Rabbat, her father, and Dr. Giovanni at their home in Bangladesh.

Dr. Giovanni gave them some herbs and home remedies.

When we arrived back at Rabbat's home, I read the first chapters of this book to Reshma, Rabbat, and her family.

They listened attentively, reliving every detail and sharing more context.

"You will share our story?" Reshma asked.

"Yes, I think it will bring so many people hope," I said. "I imagine they will feel inspired to know that if you follow your heart and listen to the inner voice that comes from God, or you may call it the spirit or Allah, deeper healing like this is possible. Your story has changed my life, and I hope it will also help many others."

"We were at the point of desperation," Reshma said. "But there was a solution, there was hope. Please tell our story so more can know. It is a miracle; Rabbat is with us."

Dr. Giovanni's phone rang. It was Dr. Naram asking to speak with Rabbat first and then Reshma, who teared up as she spoke to him. I remembered the first time I saw her, and how different these tears were than the ones I saw on her cheeks then. Finally, she handed the phone to me.

"Now you know," Dr. Naram said slowly, "how I can sleep so well at night. You have seen some cases, but think how many there have been in the last thirty-six years of my work, and in the thousands of years of my lineage. It is not me, I know that, but I am grateful to be a part of it. I thank my master every day for teaching me these secrets, so I can be of service to others."

"You help people deeply," I said, reflecting back on what I'd seen and experienced since meeting Dr. Naram, and how much I learned about the human heart, about hope, about healing and resilience. "I wish more people could meet you, Dr. Naram."

"Remember, I wasn't the one who helped Rabbat, it was Dr. Giovanni. I did not even need to be there, when the ancient healing principles and methods were. And it was the faith of her mother, Reshma, which created the transformation. Anyone who has that kind of a burning desire and faith can learn to use these ancient secrets to benefit and transform their lives. In a way, I suppose you could call them self-healing secrets."

Before saying goodbye, Dr. Naram said, "Getting health and life back is one thing. Now the real question for Rabbat, for you Clint, for me, and for everyone is this: 'What do we do with our life while we have life in us?' What I want most for you is to discover what you want and how to manifest your dreams into reality." Before ending the phone call, Dr. Naram said with certainty, "When you truly understand the principles of this ancient science, Clint, it will change everything."

Only now, after more than ten years since first meeting Dr. Naram, can I see just how true that statement turned out to be.

Your Journal Notes

What are the most valuable insights, questions, or realizations that came to you while reading this book?

_____

_____

_____

_____

_____

_____

What, if anything, would you like to commit to doing differently in your life from this point forward?

_____

_____

_____

_____

_____

_____

Mystical Miracles of Love

"When the student is ready, the teacher appears.
When the student is truly ready, the teacher disappears."

–Lao Tzu

You've now read this book which tells the story of my first year with Dr. Naram. My journey with him continued for more than ten years, and you are now a part of it.

I started this book by saying, "You are not reading these words by accident... I believe you were led to this book at this point in time for a specific reason."

Do you know your reason yet? What has reading it done for you? I'd love to support you in your journey, wherever your path leads you now. In the Author's Note after this, I share with you a gift which includes invaluable resources I've compiled for you.

Before that, however, I want to share from my heart to your heart an experience that happened just before publishing this book. It speaks volumes about how precious every day of our lives are.

On Feb 19, 2020, I received the heartbreaking news informing me that I needed to rush back to Mumbai immediately, as Dr. Naram had unexpectedly passed away. At first, I couldn't believe it. Even if doctors had declared him dead, I thought he would find some way to escape it.

Dr. Naram had been traveling alone on a trip to both Nepal and Dubai. Usually, I went with him on every tour, but this time he had asked me to stay in India and attend a conference in Delhi. I received messages and calls from him every day while he was traveling, sharing some of his new clarity and discoveries. For example, he enthusiastically told me he saw twenty-seven major trends and challenges the world was heading towards, including the virus pandemic, and how the ancient healing secrets could help with each of them. As we discussed the coming challenges, I felt so grateful that whatever we faced, we had Dr. Naram and these ancient secrets to help us.

One of the last patients who saw Dr. Naram in Dubai, told me, "He was full of vibrant energy, touching our hearts, bringing us hope, and making us all laugh. We never thought it could be our last time with him."

When Dr. Naram was on board his flight back to India, he called home and spoke with his son, Krushna, his wife, Smita, and some visitors in his home, Inga and Jack Canfield (Jack is the co-author of the *Chicken Soup for the Soul* series). They had come to India, like

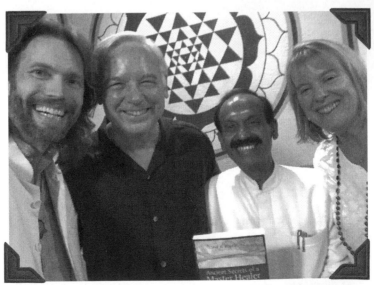

Dr. Clint G. Rogers with Jack and Inga Canfield and Dr. Naram.
Photo taken the day before Dr. Naram left India for Nepal.

my dad, to experience a month of a panchakarma wellness retreat. The conversation Dr. Naram had with each of them was light and jovial, and full of love.

Once his flight landed in Mumbai, Dr. Naram called Vinay to say he had arrived safely, and asked if the car was there to pick him up. Somewhere between getting off the plane and going through customs, airport officials reported that Dr. Naram suddenly collapsed. He was immediately rushed in an ambulance to the hospital, where they declared him dead on arrival. Without doing an autopsy, they claimed the cause of death was heart failure, and the body was burned less than 12 hours later. In India it is customary to burn the body very quickly, as there is a belief that then the spirit can be more free to move on.

My mind couldn't make sense of anything that was happening. I was with Dr. Naram in Berlin only a couple of months earlier, when a German doctor ran several tests on his heart and had found his heart to be functioning in the normal range for a man his age. That is all the more reason why I found the news hard to believe.

Since I was still in Delhi, I rushed immediately back to Mumbai. My body numb and shocked, I took a taxi straight from the airport to the crematory. As we passed through congested traffic, painful thoughts kept running through my head. "This can't be true. He seemed so invincible! How could this have happened to my mentor, my teacher, my friend?! We need him!" My taxi pulled up right after Dr. Naram's family had arrived with his body for the burning.

As I walked through the crowd of people toward his body, I connected eye-to-eye with each person, and a flood of memories came. I knew their stories, and I knew how deeply Dr. Naram had loved and helped each one. I couldn't hold back the tears. As the reality of his passing sunk in more, I felt the devastating burden of loss—for those who knew him and for all those who now would not be able to meet him.

For the last years of Dr. Naram's life, I'd been like his shadow. Now his brother, students, and closest friends were hugging me, many saying how grateful they were for what I had done in collecting the stories and secrets of Dr. Naram's life.

It had been difficult enough to contain my emotions, so imagine what it felt like when I walked up next to Dr. Naram's son. When we first met, Krushna was ten years old. Now he was twenty, and had been one of my best friends for years. Only a month prior I'd seen Krushna speak in front of an audience of 300,000 people and touch everyone's heart. We'd traveled to the USA, Nepal, and Europe together, experiencing so much, and yet we never anticipated this moment. As I put my arm around his shoulder to support him, a fresh stream of tears found their way down my cheeks.

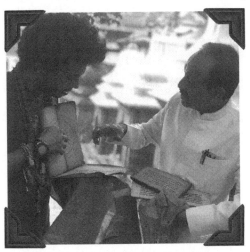

Dr. Naram teaching his son, Krushna, secret principles behind the functioning of the ancient Siddha-Veda remedies.

Then it was Krushna who comforted me. He spoke to me and to others near in a calm and clear voice. "You know he is not his body. His body is just like a shirt, and now he has gone to get a new shirt. His death is not to be mourned, but his life is to be celebrated."

I was in awe. How was Krushna so grounded, wise, and loving, even in this most difficult situation? He walked from person to person holding their hands, sometimes putting his hand on their heart or around their shoulder, comforting each person he touched.

While witnessing this, I felt like I heard Dr. Naram's voice in my head, with bittersweet words coming to memory. Dozens of times in the years we spent together, whenever he got excited that I had just learned one of the key secrets of his lineage, Dr. Naram joyfully told me, "I'm so glad you finally learned this thing! Now you can share it with Krushna and others in the future." Watching Krushna now, however, I felt like there was a lot I wanted to learn from him.

Throughout the last ten years, I'd taken many pictures and videos of Dr. Naram around the world, documenting his healing work and mission. Out of habit, I pulled out my phone to capture some of the moments at the crematory as well, until it was too much. It felt so surreal taking pictures of his body, lying peacefully still on a plank of wood and covered in garlands of flowers. I slid my phone back into my pocket and decided to just be present. Looking at him lying there, I wanted badly for him to get up, tell us a story that would inspire us and make us laugh and help us feel like everything was going to be OK. But he just laid there, eyes closed and motionless.

After some rituals, the men in Dr. Naram's family surrounded his body and picked it up. Dr. Naram's older brother, Vidyutt, motioned me to join as one of the family members in carrying the body. We walked the body around the stack of wood several times, eventually placing it on top.

Soon after, Krushna held a flaming piece of wood out in front of him, igniting Dr. Naram's final resting bed. As I watched the flames begin to rise and crackle around his body, I reflected on all the years of seeing him so full of life and healing energy. We would stay at the clinic until sometimes three or four in the morning, and he would have even more energy than at the beginning of the day.

As Krushna stood next to the burning body, I remembered a priceless moment from only a few weeks before with them both. The last long day of clinic in India ended after midnight and we all thought we were going home. Dr. Naram, however, surprised his students and Krushna by taking us all out to the roads of Mumbai. The trunk of his car was full of blankets, and we spent the next couple of hours finding homeless men, women, and children on the streets and covered them while they were sleeping.

Although it was not the first time we had done this, I wondered why at the end of a very long clinic, Dr. Naram would want to take us all to do this. He told me, "Clint, even though our day at clinic is over, these people are still suffering in the cold. We must help them. When I was young and got kicked out of my home, I had to sleep the first night on the streets, and I remember how cold and lonely I was. During the night a stranger put a blanket on me. I only noticed when I woke up. I'll never know who that was, but I blessed them, and committed in the future to help others who may be in need like I was." I imagined how grateful he must have been, kicked out of his home and sleeping on the streets, to be touched by love in a critical moment when he needed it the most. "When you do this kind of a thing, anonymously, with no need of anything in return, ultimately, God blesses you with a feeling no amount of money can buy," he said.

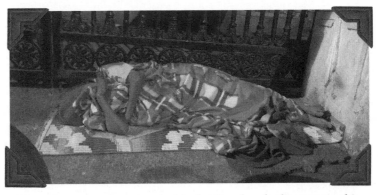

A homeless person hugging the blanket Krushna had just put on him.

As a blanket of fire now warmed Dr. Naram's body, I remembered in the years I was with him all the hundreds of blankets we placed on people sleeping on the street corners and under bridges, and the looks on the faces of some of the people who woke up to the kindness of strangers. Wherever I went with Dr. Naram, he always had food or money in his car or pocket to give to anyone who came up to him in need—people, animals, anyone. He said, "My master taught me that *Atithi Devo Bhava.* (guests are equivalent to God) is not just a concept, but a way of life." I saw it was true for him. Dr. Naram always had something to give homeless children that came to knock on his car window, or biscuits to give hungry street dogs that crossed his path. It didn't matter to him how late it was, or how much he had already done.

That night, as we drove around placing blanket after blanket on people, I saw Dr. Naram getting happier and happier. As Dr. Naram and I watched Krushna walk across the street to place blankets on a sleeping homeless woman and her children, he sighed and told me, "I want Krushna to know that the greater a man is, the more humble he should become. People don't come to me from around the world because I'm a 'great doctor'. They come because I love them, because I understand them, and because I find solutions to their burning problems. When I see Krushna do this with so much love, I feel so proud. I realize I do not have to worry about him anymore, as he knows there is no better blessing than when you can really love and serve people who are in need."

The Death of a Master, The Birth of a Movement

In my first radio interview after Dr. Naram's passing, the host asked me a question I think so many people around the world were asking themselves. "Dr. Naram's master had lived so long, yet Dr. Naram was so young, only 65, when he passed away. How could this be?"

I started by replying to the radio host, "Some things we may never know the reason..." I suppose it's likely we all had taken for granted and assumed Dr. Naram would live longer. But in the end, even with the ancient secrets, we are all mortal. We don't know when our last breath will be. I thought about my experience with Rabbat in the ICU, noticing the air coming in and out of my lungs, realizing that every single breath is a gift.

As I paused to breathe, I recalled beautiful words my sister told me; "The truth about death is that no one can hold it off forever. And more important than how he died is instead how he lived, and how he loved."

In a flash, my mind reflected on all those Dr. Naram had loved: his patients, his friends, and his family. I thought of many of his students that he loved, not yet mentioned in this book, like Sandhya from

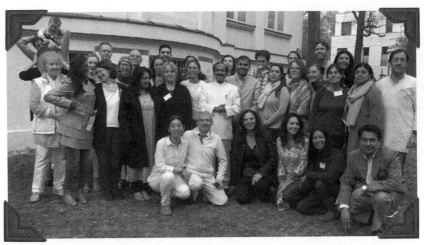

*Dr. Naram with his students for the Ancient Traditions of Healing
certification course at a university in Berlin.*

Japan; Drs. Mehta, Sahaj, Pranita and others from India; Alvaro
and Videh from Italy; Sarita, Sascha and Rebecca from England;
Jutta from Austria; Radu from Romania; Dr. Siddiqui from Bangladesh; Richard from Norway; Dipika from Australia; Suyogi, Elinor,
Dubravka, Jonas, Mira, Anne, Pooja, Moksha and Shital from Germany; and so many others. I was grateful for all the other doctors
and practitioners he had taught in Italy, and the many others from
around the world who had participated in Dr. Naram's certification
course through the university in Berlin. Over more than thirty-six
years he'd taught so many students, and I was honored to be one
of them.

I then thought of Dr. Naram's wife, Dr. Smita, who had been
with him for so many years, running the entire Panchakarma clinic
in Mumbai as well as training other doctors. I thought of his son,
Krushna, and how Dr. Naram was so proud of the man he was
becoming. Krushna had been trained in pulse healing since he was
old enough to sit on his papa's lap, and already his ability to help
people was inspiring.

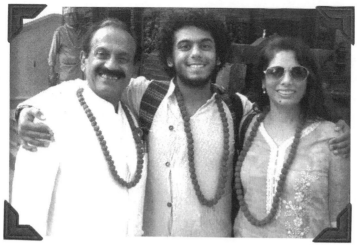

Dr. Naram, Krushna, and Smita in Nepal.

I also thought about this book you are reading now, and all the other people who would learn about the ancient healing science through it. In everything, I saw how the death of this master was not the end, as he had already put into place the birth of a movement.

The peaceful feeling in my heart inspired the rest of my response. To the radio host, I replied with a Lao Tzu quote my friend Amrutha had just sent to me. It seemed to resonate as being true in this moment: "When the student is ready the teacher appears. When the student is TRULY ready, the teacher disappears."

Manifestations of Mystical Miracles of Love

Only some time later, I realized the problem with the word "disappear" is it gives off the impression that if a person has left their body, that is the end. But what if something else is the truth? What if Dr. Naram never actually disappeared, but is more with us now than ever?

In the time since Dr. Naram's passing, many people have reported mystical things happening. Several spiritual leaders told me in almost the exact same words, "The universe/God must have had a very big need to have taken Dr. Naram so quickly. For a soul that is a master like him to depart the body like that, there must be an important reason. Now that Dr. Naram is not constrained by a body, he can enjoy going about his healing work in a greater way than ever before."

I've noticed that even if we aren't fully aware of Dr. Naram's presence in spirit, there are mystical, magical things happening all the time since his passing. Many of which, by the way they are done, seem clearly to be done by his hand. Can you just imagine his smile from the other side as he continues to help orchestrate miracles?

As one example of this, already dozens of people, including Krushna, Smita, my friend Mina (who was visiting India at the time), have told me about remarkable appearances Dr. Naram made to them since his passing. Usually it was in a dream, but sometimes it was while the person was awake. Each appearance conveyed an important healing message or experience for that person.

You were also attracted to reading this book, and his story, for a reason. In light of that, I imagine that Dr. Naram feels connected to you, and perhaps you will feel his presence too. Though I personally have not seen him since he passed, I did have one quite unexplainable experience I want to share with you.

On the morning after the prayer service for Dr. Naram at about 5:30am I woke up feeling especially lost and lonely. A dark cloud of an oncoming depression started to cast over my mind. It was still dark outside, too, but I couldn't sleep. So, I got out of bed, put my shoes on and went for a walk. Twenty minutes into my aimless wander, I suddenly became aware that someone was following me. At first it startled me, but then I saw it was a dog. He had brown legs, head, and tail, with black fur on his back, almost like a coat. His belly and a good portion of his nose were white. When I stopped to look at him, he stopped to look at me. When I continued walking, he followed closely behind. I was bewildered. Why was this dog following me?

I didn't have any food with me, and my hands were empty. It was a long walk and no matter which way I turned or what path I took, this dog stayed with me. It was both amusing and confusing.

Breaking through my sadness came this thought; I remembered Dr. Naram always had something for dogs or anyone that came to him. I heard his voice in my mind, "Atithi Devo Bhava." (Treat the unexpected guest as if god/goddess himself/herself has come to visit you.) As the sun rose and shops opened, I bought some biscuits for this unexpected visitor, as he patiently sat on the ground and waited for me. However, when I placed the biscuits on the ground in front of him, the dog sniffed them and then looked back up at me without taking a bite or even so much as licking them.

Now I was even more perplexed. If he was not hungry, then what did he want from me?

I kept walking and sure enough, he got up and followed me, leaving the biscuits behind for another dog or lucky animal. By now, whatever sadness I had felt was gone, and in its place was a playful awe at what was happening. As we walked together, I started remembering many things Dr. Naram had taught me which, in light of his passing, impacted me in new ways. Feeling the value of all that and the magic of the appearance of this dog, I pulled out my phone and recorded a Facebook live video to share with others who might also be suffering with the news of Dr. Naram's passing.

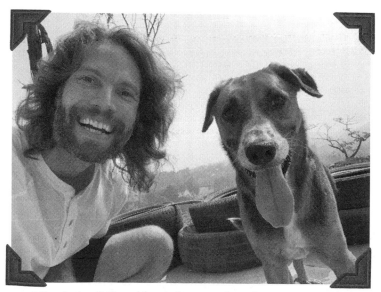

Miracle dog, Milo, and me after one of our first walks together.

The response from the video was phenomenal. People all over the world left comments remarking on the way in which it helped them in their healing process. Immediately after, I met with Krushna, who upon seeing the dog also had memories come back to him. We got excited by the insights they brought.

That evening, however, I was faced with a challenge. I didn't know what to do with this dog that would bark or whine if I left him outside the door. Eventually, I decided to truly treat this unexpected guest as if God himself had come. I wouldn't leave God outside to sleep on the street, would I? So, I cautiously let the dog in. I was pleasantly surprised that he did not scratch any furniture or pee on the floor. Thank you, God. He just laid on the ground in whatever room I went to and looked up at me. When it was time to sleep, he would only stop whining if he could lay on the floor right next to my bed, with my hand on his head.

There is so much that I could say about this divine dog. I now call him Bhairava (which is a divine manifestation of God in the form of a dog) or miracle Milo (because I found him when I was at *my low*, but his appearance brought me to *my love*). His magical appearance sparked deep healing. His presence has shown me that we truly are never alone. There are signs of divine love all around us, and all we need to do is look for them.

When I first heard about Dr. Naram's passing, I thought, "Is this the end? What comes next?" The healing Milo brought me is such a great reminder that his passing is NOT the end. Just that the story took a different turn than we expected or wanted. I have many more stories from the past with Dr. Naram to share with you, but Milo also taught me that many more stories will come in the future.

What I'm very excited about is that you, now, are part of the continuing story. I'm very curious what part you will play in the rest of the story, and what part of that story will we experience together. My time with Milo reminded me that we are all in this together, and none of us is ever truly alone.

Along those lines, here is one final experience I will share with you. On the second day Milo was with me, my friend Mina and I needed to go to the clinic. I didn't know what to do with Milo. When I called an Uber, Milo followed me to the car. As soon as Mina and I got in the car, Milo jumped right in after us and plopped down on my lap. The Uber driver did not look happy but, thankfully, decided to drive us anyway.

Milo sat on my lap for the entire 35-minute drive. Mina remarked how strange and interesting it was that a street dog would do this. When we arrived at the clinic, Milo jumped out of the car and immediately started wagging his tail. I was nervous to let him walk with me in the hallways of the facility, but he wouldn't have it any other way. I justified it in my mind by thinking that since many people would bring their animals to see Dr. Naram, I assumed the staff would be used to it. Once at the clinic, another amazing thing happened, and I too captured it on a Facebook live video.

On the second floor of the building, the dog left me and went straight to the office where Dr. Naram would see patients. A staff member opened the door, and we all were completely surprised when Milo went right in, looked up at the picture of Dr. Naram and Smita with the Dalai Lama, then looked at the chair where Dr. Naram would sit. Then Milo sat down right in front of the desk as if he belonged there. Tears started to fall down the cheeks of the staff who came in

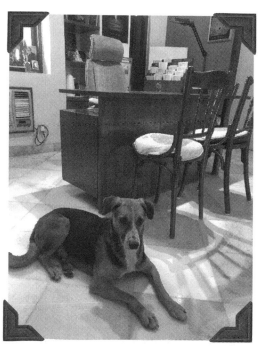

Milo, sitting on the floor in front of Dr. Naram's desk. to witness the mystical

unfolding. Even I had to go back to watch my Facebook live video to see if it really happened that way, or if I just imagined it.

As many of the staff came to see and take pictures with Milo, the whole experience renewed a sense of awe and wonder in all of us. Soon after, I closed the doors to the office and Mina, Milo, and I sat there for a while. Mina and I closed our eyes to meditate and, in the silence, a memory came of one of my first times in that room—from ten years ago when I first visited India with Alicia.

Right next to where Milo was now sitting, Dr. Naram had pulled me aside out of the crowd of people who were waiting. I thought it was strange that he had singled me out to talk and so I curiously listened as he spoke, "I don't know why, Clint, but I believe in you." He paused. "Perhaps there is a reason you are here. I have a strong feeling you will do something great in your life, that you will be successful in doing the things you want to do." With his hand on my arm, he looked me in my eyes and said, "The main question is, what do you want?"

As this memory came, a big smile spread across my face, breaking up the stream of tears flowing down my cheeks.

And that is the question, dear one, that I'll also leave with you now.

What do you want?

What Next?

Live as if you were to die tomorrow.
Learn as if you were to live forever.
–Mahatma Gandhi

So what is next for you? People ask me, "Clint, now that Dr. Naram has passed, where do I go to experience the ancient secrets?"

Dr. Naram taught me that eighty percent of the time there are simple things you can do to heal yourself. You just need to apply certain principles and have a little support. How do you discover more?

Register now at the free membership website:
www.MyAncientSecrets.com/Belong

1. You'll get links to video trainings by Dr. Naram, myself, and others, matching up to each chapter, with home remedies, herbal remedies, marmaa, and diet secrets that can help you.
2. If you want to talk with someone in person about your situation, you'll see how.

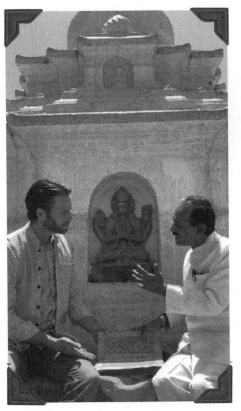

Dr. Naram and me at the exact same place where his master taught him.

3. You'll get links for any events or training (live and online), and you can discover how to invite me or someone else to speak at your event.

4. You'll find out more about a workbook that goes along with this book, called *Discover Yourself: Applying Ancient Secrets That Can Change Your Life* (which includes advanced content not found in this book). It helps you personalize and apply this time-tested wisdom, for your physical, mental, emotional, and spiritual well-being.

5. As a fun bonus, we created a game for you called *30-Days to Unlocking Your Ancient Secret Power*. It can help you, as you play, to experience more vibrant health, unlimited energy, and peace of mind.

6. You'll instantly be connected with a community of people who want to make a difference on this planet, and you become part of our family.

I'm excited to see what happens in your life when you join us.

Note: As far as I know, this is the first book published in English about Dr. Naram's ancient healing secrets. I was not asked to write or paid to write this book by anyone. I felt inspired to write it. This book is not the definitive work on either Dr. Naram or Siddha-Veda, but simply my perspective. I hope it captures and honors the vibrant and dynamic nature of this special man and master healer, as well as the emotions of those who shared their stories with me. Some of the people I interviewed asked to remain anonymous, so I have changed their names. The rest have given permission to share their stories publicly and, in some cases, said I could share their contact information with anyone who wants it. In a few of the cases I made composite characters to help the people remain anonymous and to maintain the story's fluidity. All of the people who shared their experiences expressed a hope that they might help inspire others when they need it most. I've done a follow-up interview or video with many people mentioned in this book, such as Rabbat, so you can find out what is happening in their lives now. You can find these on the MyAncientSecrets.com membership website, too.

Special Thanks & Acknowledgments: The list of people to thank is so long, I've needed to put it on the website, MyAncientSecrets. com. For all those who have helped in any way with sharing stories, reviewing, editing, and giving feedback on this book, I give a deep bow of gratitude for you. The blessing of your love is felt in each page of this book.

Next Book: Because this book details only a handful of the countless stories and home remedies I have captured, I'm already working on the next book in the series which includes more life-changing stories and secrets. When you join the membership website, you'll see how you can be updated when the next book is published. MyAncientSecrets.com/Belong.

Your Journey: Mahatma Gandhi stated that all of us are interconnected. Whenever one person suffers, we all suffer to that same extent. Conversely, when one person is helped, all of humanity is lifted to that same degree. If this book has helped you in any way, I invite you to leave a five-star review on Amazon.com, as well as share what you've learned with those you love. For every single life you touch and improve, all of humanity benefits to that same extent.

This book is not actually about Dr. Naram, and never has been. And it is not about me, either. You may never meet either of us or follow this method of healing.

This book is about *You*, and always has been. It's about you seeing the divine inside yourself, which can guide you to the exact experiences, teachers, and healing which are perfect for you. My hope is that as a result of joining the journey of reading this book you will feel more love, an increased desire to take better care of yourself, and more awe at the miracle of all of life.

You truly are a beautiful, unique, and brilliant part of the divine tapestry of existence. All of life is happening *for* you, not *to* you.

And you *are* being guided. As evidence of this reality—you are reading these words right now.

You may even have had guided inspiration while reading this book about some actions you should take, and I'd encourage you to do those things. Or perhaps a thought came of someone you would like to share this book with. You never know who needs that gift of love right now.

I do have one final small request for you.

I invite you to pause for a few minutes now, and either close your eyes, or write free-flow style in the space below.

Take some time now and write down here each moment, person, and experience you remember that has contributed to your life and for which you feel grateful for:

_____

_____

_____

_____

_____

_____

Look at your list again now, and as you read each one, in your heart say "thank you" to life. Then at the end say "thank you" for the gift of being you, exactly who you are, exactly where you are, in this exact moment in time. Thank you.

Just as I was guided to help my father, and many people and experiences were perfectly placed in my path to lead me to where I am now, the truth is you have been guided, too. By love. Trust you will continue to be guided, by love, to exactly what is right for you.

And I hope you always remember that whatever problems you may face, each one has a solution. Even better, as Dr. Naram said, "Every problem or challenge has within it the seeds of equal or greater opportunity."

Namaste,
Dr. Clint G. Rogers

P.S. I'd love to stay in touch with you, to hear your story of how you were led to this book and your experiences from reading it. You can connect with me on Facebook, Instagram, or email me at DrClint@MyAncientSecrets.com.

APPENDIX

Guide to New Words

Aam (or ama) = toxins

Agni = ancient term used to describe digestive fire or power

Allopathy, or **Allopathic Medicine** = a system of medical practice that aims to combat disease by use of remedies (as drugs or surgery) producing effects different from or incompatible with those produced by the disease being treated (*Merriam-Webster Medical Dictionary* definition).

Amrapali = considered to be one of the most beautiful women ever born; using ancient Siddha-Veda youth and beauty secrets she learned from Jivaka, she maintained her youth and beauty so much that the young king, who already had a young and beautiful wife, fell in love with Amrapali, even though she was over twenty years older than him.

Ancient healing = not about "fighting diseases" but about creating balance in the body, often through purification from toxins, through which the body heals itself.

MyAncientSecrets.com Free Membership Website = a gift to you for reading this book, and a resource for learning how to immediately apply these ancient healing secrets in your own life. Start here: www.MyAncientSecrets.com/Belong.

Ancient Traditions of Healing (ATH) = the two-year certification course in the ancient healing methods of Dr. Naram and Siddha-Veda, originally offered through a university in Berlin and now spreading to other universities around the world.

'Atithi Devo Bhava' = Indian saying that means you treat any guest, whoever it is and however inconvenient their visit may be, as if God himself has come to your home. In the healing lineage of Siddha-Veda, they take this saying very much to heart, considering every person who comes as a manifestation of God.

Atmiyata (pronounced *Aht-me-yah-tah*) = powerful life principle taught by Hariprasad Swamijii and practiced by members of the Yogi Divine Society: no matter how someone treats you, you can respond with love and respect.

Ayurveda = science of life; over 5,000 year-old medical science from India that focuses both on overcoming sickness, and what kind of lifestyle helps with prevention of disease in the first place.

Blocks (physical, mental, emotional, relationship, spiritual, financial, etc.) = where life gets stuck, then starts to stink (and get difficult). Deeper healing comes when we can recognize and remove the blocks in a safe, long-term way.

Buddha = spiritual master originally named Sidhartha Gautama, who was born in India approximately 2,500 years ago; known for giving up a life of privilege in a palace to follow, and later teach, a path to enlightenment.

Conscious, subconscious, superconscious = three levels of consciousness, which are activated through Marmaa Shakti.

Dard Mukti (pronounced *dahrd mook-tea*) = *Dard* means "pain," and *Mukti* means "freedom from"; ancient healing secrets that help relieve different kinds of joint or muscle discomfort.

Dis-ease = how Dr. Naram speaks about imbalances — that there is an imbalance, creating un-ease or dis-ease, and when you remove the block and rebalance the system, the ease in your life returns.

Deeper healing = going beyond the surface symptoms to resolve the root cause of a problem on physical, mental, emotional, and spiritual levels.

Doshas = representations in the body of the elements that exist in nature (i.e. *kapha*=earth/water, *vata*=wind/ether, *pitta*=fire); when our doshas are in balance, we are healthy, when they are out of balance, the imbalance creates dis-ease.

Ghee = clarified butter made by cooking out the solids from milk, then used in cooking and for medicinal purposes.

Gurudwara = place of worship for people of Sikh faith.

Jivaka = master healer who lived around the year 500 B.C. Known as the first master of the Siddha-Veda lineage, he was also the personal physician for Lord Buddha; Amrapali, considered to be one of the most beautiful women in the world; and the Indian King Bimbisāra. He learned, recorded in ancient manuscripts, and passed on to his students the secret knowledge he discovered about achieving vibrant health, unlimited energy, and peace of mind at any age.

Kapha = the *dosha*, or life element, related to earth/water.

Karmayog, bhaktiyog, and gyanyog = different paths to moksha, a state of enlightenment or fulfillment (i.e. path of meditation, path of prayer, path of success in business or in battle).

Marmaa Shakti = an ancient technology of deeper transformation, working on all levels—body, mind, emotions, and spirit. Knowingly or unknowingly, everyone is programmed by society. Marmaa is an ancient technology for reprogramming yourself to align your life with your true purpose. It can help remove blocks and rebalance your system. Not only can physical pain reduce or disappear, this ancient technology can also help you achieve whatever it is that you want in life.

Moksha = state of enlightenment or fulfillment.

Namaste (pronounced *Nah-mah-stay*) or **Namaskar** (pronounced *Nah-mah-skar*) = greeting in India made by pressing hands together in front of the heart, meaning "the divine god/goddess in me bows to the divine god/goddess in you, and I honor that place where you and I are one."

Pakoda (pronounced *pah-koh-dah*) = an Indian dish similar to onion rings, which Dr. Naram used to get rid of my intense headache and demonstrate the principle that everything can be a medicine or a poison depending on how/when/where you use it.

Panchakarma or asthakarma (pronounced *pahnch-ah-kahr-mah* and *ahst-ah-kahr-mah*) = a multiprocess cleansing and rebuilding of the body's core systems, one of Siddha-veda's six keys of deeper healing. *Karma* means "action," and *pancha* means "five." So panchakarma consists of five actions to remove toxins from, or cleanse, the body. In asthakarma, there are eight actions, or three additional steps, to cleanse, purify, and rebalance the body from the inside out.

Pankaj Naram (pronounced *Pahn-kahj Nah-rahm*) = the master healer (Dr. Naram) referred to in this book, born May 4, 1955, and left his body February 19, 2020.

Pitta = the *dosha*, or life element, related to fire.

Pulse healing = an ancient method of diagnosis whereby the healer touches the pulse of the patient and, based on the way in which the pulse is jumping, is able to determine what imbalances and blocks are in the body, and how they impact physical, mental, emotional, and spiritual health.

Seva (pronounced *say-vah*) = translated means "service."

Shakti = defined as "power"; or the divine power to do things or create things. According to Dr. Naram, this power is already in you, and *marmaa shakti* is an ancient instrument which helps to bring it out—working with the other keys of Siddha-Veda to help people experience vibrant health.

Siddha-Veda (or **Siddha-Raharshayam**) = healing lineage or school of thought with secrets for deeper healing that go a step beyond Ayurveda, taught from master to student, with secrets or "technology" for helping you discover, achieve, and enjoy what you want.

> 95 percent of people on this planet do not know what they want;
>
> 3 percent know what they want but can't achieve it;
>
> 1 percent know what they want, achieve it, but then do not enjoy it.
>
> Only 1 percent of people know what they want, achieve it, and enjoy it.

Siddha-Veda's Six Keys of Deeper Healing = diet, home remedies, herbal remedies, marmaa shakti, lifestyle, and panchakarma/asthakarma. These help keep people looking and feeling young at any age.

Vaidya = a Sanskrit word meaning "physician," used in India to refer to a person who practices the indigenous Indian systems of medicine.

Vata = the *dosha,* or life element, related to wind/ether.

Yagna (pronounced *Yahg-nah*) = a type of a ritual with a specific objetive.

Comparison of Allopathy (Modern Western Medicine), Ayurveda, and Siddha-Veda

	Allopathy	Ayurveda	Siddha-Veda
How old?	200+ years old, first named in 1810	5,000+ years old	2,500+ years old
Who started?	Samuel Hahnemann (1755–1843) coined the term "Allopathy" to distinguish it from "Homeopathy"	One of the original scholars, Sushruta, said he was taught this method of medicine from Dhanvantari, incarnated as king of Varanasi at the time	Jivaka (physician for Buddha and other famous contemporaries)
How passed on?	Medical schools & residency	Books, universities, and practica	Apprenticeship of master to student, in an unbroken lineage
What is its basic focus?	Treatment of symptoms of disease with medications and surgeries; breaks down body into parts, with specialists focusing on individual parts	Defined as "science of life," focused on proper living which also helps prevent or overcome disease (applied on an individualized basis depending on the person's dosha constitution) — sees interconnection of all parts of body, mind, and emotions and creates remedies that understand this	Helping people achieve vibrant health, unlimited energy and peace of mind (applied on an individualized basis depending on the person's dosha constitution) — sees interconnection of all parts of body, mind, and emotions and creates remedies that understand this; also helps people discover what they want, achieve what they want, and enjoy what they have achieved

What are diagnosis methods?	Using external machines to capture measurable data (e.g., temperature, blood pressure, blood sugar levels, etc.)	Using direct perception of physician (e.g., through pulse, tongue, observation of urine, etc.)	Using direct perception of physician (e.g., through pulse and other methods based on the situation)
What are main instruments/ methods of healing?	Medications and surgery	Herbal formulas, home remedies, diet, lifestyle, panchakarma	6 instruments, or "keys," of healing: home remedies, diet, marmaa shakti, herbal formulas, panchakarma/ asthakarma, lifestyle
Verification methods?	Double-blind studies (which isolate variables and test them in a controlled environment over a period of months or years)	Impact of remedy on immediate health, and observed over extended period of time, with a variety of people, over thousands of years	Impact of remedy on immediate health, and observed over extended period of time, with a variety of people, over thousands of years
What are strengths?	Often can be a quick fix	Focused on long-term benefit	Focused on deeper healing and long-term benefit; always high-quality herbs that are heavy-metal–free
What are downsides?	Often there are negative side effects of the treatments; also you often need to see a specialist and either have insurance or pay a lot out of pocket	Often takes time, effort, lifestyle change, and patience to see results; varying quality of physician or herbs; sometimes heavy metals found in herbs	Long wait to see a physician, because of high demand; often takes time, effort, lifestyle change, and patience to see results; herbs are priced at premium due to quality

*On MyAncientSecrets.com, you can find more discussion on the distinctions between the above three methodologies as well as other forms of traditional and 'alternative' healing.

My Journal Notes (Bonus Secret for You)
AMRAPALI'S SECRET

Three Ancient Secrets for Supporting Women of Any Age (from 15 to age 60+) for Optimal Hormone Levels*

1) Home Remedy—Dr. Naram's Amrapali's Secret Home Remedy

      250g Fennel Powder
      250g Cumin Powder
      50g Ajwain Powder
      50g Black Salt
      50g Dill Seeds
      25g Coriander Powder
      10g Asafoetida/Hing Powder

Mix all ingredients together and divide total into 60 equal packets. (Many non-traditional ingredients may be ordered online.)

To take a packet, first soak the mixture in warm water for 30–60 minutes, and drink the entire contents. Each day you will take 4 packets like this, spread throughout the day. Continue the process for at least 6 months.

2) Marmaa Shakti for Amrapali's Secret—on the left wrist under the thumb count three points down the arm, and press that point 6 times, many times a day.

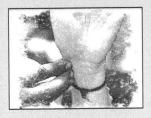 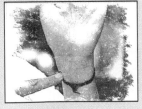

3) Herbal Remedies—there was a liquid and a tablet form of herbs to support healthy hormones in women, which included ingredients like fennel, shatavari, celery, and chastetree seeds.

*Bonus Material: You can discover more of Amrapali's secrets online in the membership site: MyAncientSecrets.com/Belong.
*Remember the medical disclaimer applies for anything in this book or online.

My Journal Notes (Bonus Secret for You)
ANCIENT SECRETS FOR IMMUNITY

In Chapter 12, Dr. Giovanni helped a hive of bees overcome a virus, in part by giving them herbs and a home remedy to boost their immunity. He got these ancient secrets from Dr. Naram who used them to help many people, giving them more vibrant health, unlimited energy, and peace of mind.

1) Diet—Boil slices of ginger root in water with 1/2 tsp turmeric powder and sip throughout the day. Avoid wheat and dairy products, as well as sour and fermented foods. Instead eat moong soup and cooked green, leafy vegetables.

2) Marmaa Shakti—On the right hand, middle finger very top portion, press 6 times, many times a day.

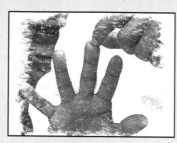

3) Home Remedy—Dr. Naram's powerful ancient home remedy to support immunity:

> 1 tsp honey
> 1/2 tsp ginger juice
> 1/2 tsp turmeric powder
> 1/4 tsp cinnamon powder
> 11-12 Tulsi (Basil) leaves
> 1/8 tsp clove powder
> 1 clove garlic (but if for religious reason you avoid garlic, then you don't need to include)
> —mix all in half a glass of warm water and take 2-4 times a day.

4) Herbal Remedies—Dr. Giovanni gave a formula of herbs for supporting immunity which included ingredients like pomegranate peel, Indian tinospora, licorice roots, holarrhena bark, andrographis roots, ginger, and holy basil leaves.

*Bonus Material: You can see this marmaa demonstrated and how to make this remedy online in the MyAncientSecrets.com membership website. Remember the medical disclaimer applies for anything in this book or online.

Herbal Formulas Mentioned in this Book*

Dr. Naram created more than 300 herbal formulas to assist people in deeper healing, which he had different names for in different countries. He created these formulations using the principles he learned from his master, from the ancient manuscripts, and from his extensive experience helping over a million people during more than 36 years. I saw how he used secret ancient processes to bring out the alchemical benefits from the combination of specific ingredients, and at the same time he utilized modern scientific facilities to ensure cleanliness, standardization, and safety. My wish is that everyone creating herbal products would do it with the same level of excellence. For any herbal supplements you use, it is wise to check if they include fresh ingredients, and ensure everything is heavy-metal free.

For educational purposes only, here is a chart listing a few of the ingredients in some of the herbal formulations mentioned in this book. It is not meant to be an exhaustive or comprehensive list. For more info on this topic, please search online or find a good teacher.

*Supporting Healthy Function of:	*Some herbal formulas may include ingredients like these:
Blood pressure	arjuna bark, Indian pennywort, boerhavia, purple tephrosia, garlic
Brain function	dwarf morning glory, gotu kola, water hyssop, shatavri, white pumpkin, celastrus seed oil
Calmness	ashwaganda, water hyssop, gotu kola, dwarf morning glory, turmeric, and licorice
Hair	sesame oil, emblic fruit, Indian penny- wort, eclipta, neem, sapindus fruit, henna leaves
Immunity	pomegranate peel, Indian tinospora, licorice roots, holarrhena bark, ginger, and holy basil leaves

Joints	winged treebine bark, Indian frankincense, chastetree leaves, ginger, and guggul gum resin
Liver	phlanthus, Indian tinospora, boerhavia, chebulic myrobalin, andrographus, caper bush
Lungs	pomegranate fruit, yellow-fruit roots, malabar nut tree leaves, licorice roots, holy basil, bael tree roots, fragrant padri tree roots
Men's hormones	sesame seeds, tribulus, Indian tinospora, ashwaganda roots, Indian kudzu rhizome, and velvet bean seeds
Muscles/joints "dard" relief	peppermint, wintergreen oil, oroxylum, pluchea, cinnamon oil, ginger, cyperus roots, turmeric, chastetree leaves
Skin	neem, turmeric, coconut oil, holy basil, sweet indrajao, cinnamon, cardamom, Indian laburnum, emblic, sal tree, and black pepper
Women's hormones	fennel, shatavari, celery, chastetree seeds, devil's cotton roots, asoka tree bark, and cumin

Note About Herbal Remedies and Home Remedies

If some ingredients or herbal formulas are not available in your country, don't worry. You still have so many other things you can do. Remember the six keys of Siddha-Veda? You can change your diet, press marmaa shakti points, or make home remedies with things in your own kitchen. Dr. Naram would often adjust the ingredients in remedies for people based on their condition, constitution, age, gender, and sometimes location too. He would also pay attention to what happened in their body as they took them, and make changes as needed. So with anything you do, listen to your body and if you can, find a great practitioner to help you. Dr. Naram would say, "The journey of a thousand miles begins with a single step. Start with whatever you have access to, and do whatever you can do." Then trust that you will be guided if anything else is needed for you.

*Regarding any remedies in this book or online, please read the medical disclaimers.

Fun Pictures and Blessings

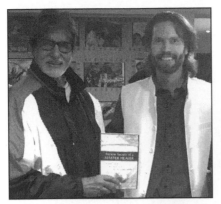

Dr. Clint G. Rogers with Bollywood Superstar Amitabh Bachchan.

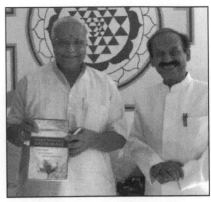

RSS leader Bhayya Joshi: "These secrets are a priceless treasure, people from India and all over the world can be proud of."

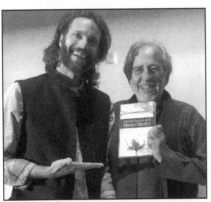

Dr. Clint G. Rogers with Dr. Bruce Lipton, Biologist & Best-selling Author.

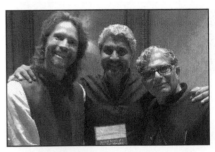

Dr. Clint G. Rogers with Poonacha Machaiah and Dr. Deepak Chopra.

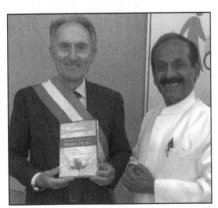

Pietro Tanzini, the Mayor of Bucine (AR), in Tuscany, Italy, refers to Dr. Naram as a "HEALING GURU."

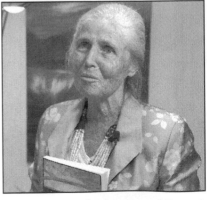

Dr. Dagmar Uecker, a respected German physician, brought Dr. Naram to her clinic in Germany every year to solve cases no one else knew how to help.

Good news! Special blessings on all who own and share this book have been given by many great saints and masters, including:

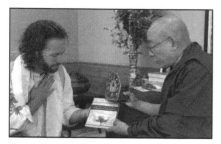

The Oracle of H.H. the 14th Dalai Lama

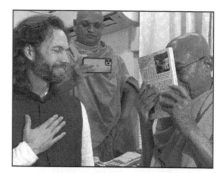

H.H. Hariprasad Swami

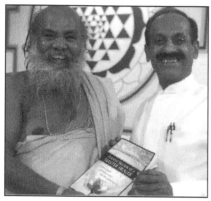

Swami Omkar Das Ji Maharaj

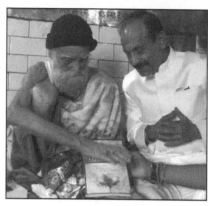

Dr. Tyaginath Aghori Baba

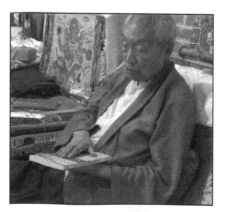

*His Eminence Namkha Drimed
Ranjam Rinpoche*

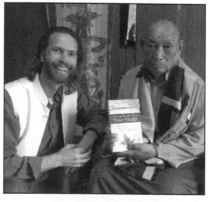

*Dr. Yeshi Dhonden,
Tibetan Medicine Healer*

***More about their blessings, and others given by spiritual leaders
of many traditions, can be found at MyAncientSecrets.com**

Letters from Saints, Scholars, and Supporters:

His Holiness Hariprasad Swami, Yogi Divine Society

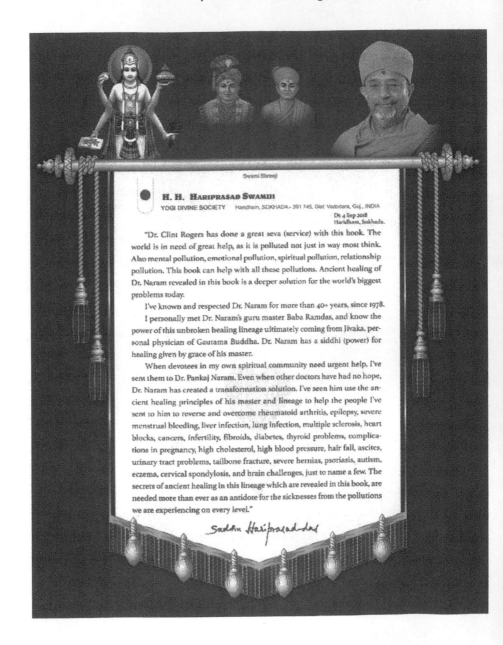

Swami Shreeji

H. H. HARIPRASAD SWAMIJI
YOGI DIVINE SOCIETY   Haridham, SOKHADA - 391 745, Dist. Vadodara, Guj., INDIA

Dt: 4 Sep 2018
Haridham, Sokhada.

"Dr. Clint Rogers has done a great seva (service) with this book. The world is in need of great help, as it is polluted not just in way most think. Also mental pollution, emotional pollution, spiritual pollution, relationship pollution. This book can help with all these pollutions. Ancient healing of Dr. Naram revealed in this book is a deeper solution for the world's biggest problems today.

I've known and respected Dr. Naram for more than 40+ years, since 1978.

I personally met Dr. Naram's guru master Baba Ramdas, and know the power of this unbroken healing lineage ultimately coming from Jivaka, personal physician of Gautama Buddha. Dr. Naram has a siddhi (power) for healing given by grace of his master.

When devotees in my own spiritual community need urgent help, I've sent them to Dr. Pankaj Naram. Even when other doctors have had no hope, Dr. Naram has created a transformation solution. I've seen him use the ancient healing principles of his master and lineage to help the people I've sent to him to reverse and overcome rheumatoid arthritis, epilepsy, severe menstrual bleeding, liver infection, lung infection, multiple sclerosis, heart blocks, cancers, infertility, fibroids, diabetes, thyroid problems, complications in pregnancy, high cholesterol, high blood pressure, hair fall, ascites, urinary tract problems, tailbone fracture, severe hernias, psoriasis, autism, eczema, cervical spondylosis, and brain challenges, just to name a few. The secrets of ancient healing in this lineage which are revealed in this book, are needed more than ever as an antidote for the sicknesses from the pollutions we are experiencing on every level."

Sadhu Hariprasaddad

ཨོཾ༎ །ཁནས་ཆུང་སྐུ་རྟེན། །

Ven. Thupten Ngodup

(The Medium of Tibet's Chief State Oracle)
Nechung Dorje Drayangling Monastery

"I am very much interested in Clint Rogers' upcoming book of Ancient Secrets of a Master Healer, because it is exactly related with Lord Buddha's teachings - 'Oh Bhikshus & Wise men, as one assays gold by rubbing, cutting & melting, so examine well my words & accept them. But not because you respect me.'

Clint Rogers has researched thoroughly about Dr. Naram's lineage of ancient techniques to cure lots of illness, especially in this century where there are so many different diseases. It is very necessary to combine both ancient and modern techniques of healing. My blessing and prayer is on this book and the millions who will read it, that their lives will be blessed with deep healing, happiness, and peace of mind."

Ven. Thupten Ngodup (Medium of Tibet's Chief State Oracle)

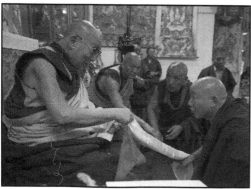

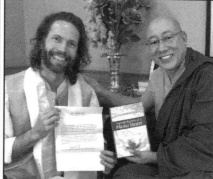

Mrs. World Supermodel & Harvard Trained Doctor

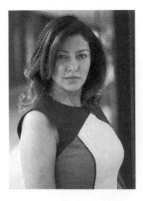

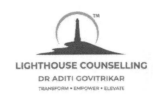

LIGHTHOUSE COUNSELLING
DR ADITI GOVITRIKAR
TRANSFORM • EMPOWER • ELEVATE

This book "Ancient Secrets of a Master Healer" by Dr. Clint G Rogers is a gift, and I want not only the people I love but every single person on this planet to read it. It is written from the heart, with timeless wisdom integrated into each engaging story—and acts like a bible of time-tested home remedies you can apply whenever you need them.

The first chapter pulled me in, and I didn't want to put it down... it was so intriguing. Simple and easy to read, it kept me on the edge of my seat always wondering, what's next?

I loved the way the stories throughout were interwoven with profound, timeless wisdom (or 'gyan' as we call it in India). It is practical and inspiring — getting me to ask important questions that make my life better—physically, emotionally and spiritually.

This book is like the Gita (or the Bible, Quran, etc) — whatever age or stage of life you are in, you will benefit from reading it. Everyone can find wisdom in it that applies to what you are experiencing at this point in your life. And every time you read it, you will find something new.

As a mother, I want every child to read the book. As a woman and model, I'm excited to apply the ancient secrets in it to look and feel younger. And as a medical doctor, I appreciate how this ancient healing science resets the body from the core. I've come to realize only ego keeps any doctor or healer from accepting the effectiveness of other forms of treatment that are different from the one that they personally practice.

With the unexpected passing of Dr. Naram, this book is needed now more than ever. As I approached the last chapter, I kept wishing the story would not end. I'm already looking forward to Dr. Clint G Rogers publishing the next book!

~ Dr. Aditi Govitrikar (Medical doctor, Harvard trained Psychologist, Mrs. World, Supermodel and Actress)

V Care Polyclinic, La Magasin, Above Roopkala Showroom, SV Road, Santacruz-54
022-26050846, 91-9820108600 | info@lighthousecounsellingcentre.com

Chairman for L&T, one of India's Most Respected Business Empires

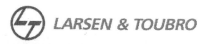 **LARSEN & TOUBRO**

A. M. Naik
Group Chairman

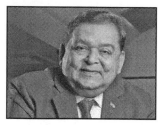

September 05, 2018

Ancient Secrets of a Master Healer

I have known Dr. Pankaj Naram for over 30 years, and seen his mission to spread healing across the world grow steadily over time.

I am delighted to have been asked to write the recommendation for this book as we share common values of integrity, hard work and most importantly, unwavering passion for whatever we may do – including propagating the relevance of ancient healing teachings in modern society.

Dr. Naram has brought to the world, ancient healing practices that had been lost over the generations. Moreover, he has helped demystify these practices and share them in a manner that can be adopted by just about anyone.

Even after touching the lives of over a million people across the globe, his devotion to his cause keeps him going from strength to strength. At an age when most people would retire, he is more passionate than ever about protecting, preserving, and bringing to the forefront ancient healing secrets (gleaned from the handwritten manuscripts of the Himalayan masters) to help heal this world more effectively.

I am sure that you will find Dr. Naram's life story as shared by university researcher Dr. Clint Rogers truly fascinating and inspiring, as you discover gems of ancient wisdom that you can apply in your daily life in this book.

I wish him all the best in his noble endeavour.

Best Regards,

A. M. Naik

A. M. Naik
Group Chairman - Larsen & Toubro

Larsen & Toubro Limited, Landmark Bldg., 'A' Wing, Suren Road, Chakala, Andheri (East), Mumbai - 400 093, INDIA
Tel: +91 22 6696 5333 Fax: +91 22 6696 5334 Email: amn@Larsentoubro.com www.Larsentoubro.com
Registered Office: L&T House, N. M. Marg, Ballard Estate, Mumbai - 400 001, INDIA CIN: L99999MH1946PLC004768

Her Holiness, Divine Premben

"Dr Pankaj Naram is a world authority in Ancient Healing Secrets.

My Guru H.H.Hariprasad Swami Maharaj (Founder - President of Yogi Divine Society) has known Dr Pankaj Naram for more than 40 years.

This book inspires one to infuse Dr Pankaj Naram's Ancient Healing Secrets in ones daily life. He helps people with diet, lifestyle, herbs, home remedies for immense energy, healthy and happy life.

I have always been touched by Dr Pankaj Naram's mission to bring the benefits into every heart and every home on earth through the Ancient Healing.

I am taking his medicine for diabetes and cholesterol and have had extraordinary results. Many Sadhvis in Bhakti Ashram (Yogi Mahila Kendra) are taking His medicines and have had incredible effect and some completely cured. Whether it be diabetes, thyroid, arthritis, joint pain, back pain asthma, and more. His Marma works wonders on people with critical condition. Dr Naram also put many of us on vegan, gluten-free diet with his herbal supplements, exercise and panchakarma. All having amazing results.

I thank Clint G Rogers for this magnificent book which every human should read."

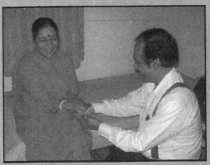

Sadhvi Suhrad

shadhvi suhrad.

President Nutritional Research Foundation
& 6-time NY Times Bestselling Author

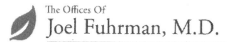

The Offices Of
Joel Fuhrman, M.D.

June 18, 2019

I appreciate Clint's friendship and comradery. He has been very interested in the extensive research I've done on how a Nutritarian diet can completely reverse health challenges like diabetes, high blood pressure, heart disease, obesity, autoimmune disease and more. My life's research, as shared through my books and PBS TV shows, demonstrates how the health problems we face are directly related to the food we eat, and that making changes in our food greatly impacts our physical, mental, and emotional health in significant ways.

Remarkable stories of people reversing all kinds of illness and diseases are not 'medical miracles'. These results are predictable when you follow certain principles. Health is your right and accessible to anyone. The problem is the toxic foods, lifestyle, and medications most people consume which put stress on our tissues year after year until they finally break down. The good news is you can heal from virtually any illness and avoid sickness to begin with, if you want to. The human body is already inherently an amazing self-repairing, self-healing machine when you simply feed it optimally with the right foods and habits.

What I love about Clint is that he is a seeker of truth with a curiosity that has led him on a unique path and mission. He has impressive knowledge of useful but generally unknown ancient healing techniques. At one point while we were in Mexico together my wife became ill with a severe digestive problem (sometimes called Montezuma's revenge). Clint quickly helped her with a remedy he knew from Dr. Naram, which we were surprised and delighted that she was well the next day. What I respect most of all is Clint's heart and powerful desire to have good will for all people. I wish him all the best with this book and in his overall mission to help humanity.

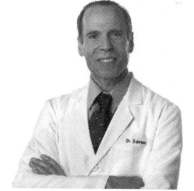

Joel Fuhrman, M.D.

President Nutritional Research Foundation

6 times NY Times Bestselling Author

4 Walter E Foran Boulevard, Suite 409, Flemington New Jersey 08822 Phone: (908) 237-0200 · Fax (908) 237-0210 · Web www.DrFuhrman.com

Other great letters can be found online.

One More Fun Story for You

In Kathmandu, Nepal, there is a temple called Swayambunath (affectionately known as the "monkey temple"). This is the place where Dr. Naram first started learning pulse healing from his master. In preparation for the publication of this book, Dr. Naram and I (Dr. Clint) went to the temple to say thank you.

At one point, I put the book down to take some pictures of it with the beautiful background... and this most unexpected event happened!

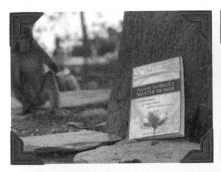
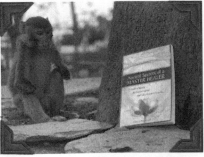

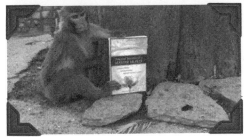

"Tantric Monkey" without hands walked over, picked up the book, & held it carefully.

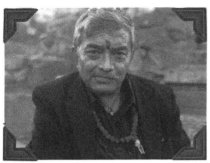

Aghori Kabiraj

Aghori Kabiraj, an informal caretaker for the over four hundred monkeys who freely roam the grounds, was in shock when he saw the photos. He said he'd never seen anything like this happen before. According to him, this was not just any monkey. Easily recognizable because he doesn't have hands, this is considered the most powerful "tantric monkey" at the temple, and a direct representative of Lord Hanuman, the monkey god.

"I don't believe my eyes," he said. "You got a miracle!" Aghori Kabiraj emphasized the unique power of this blessing. "Whatever is in this book is blessed by Hanuman, and whoever has one of these books in their home and in their lives will be blessed with that divine protection, healing, and removing any obstacles, too."

As a "Western skeptic" I honestly did not know what to make of this whole situation. Yet, as I did feel the blessing of divine power in the creation of this book, I was grateful to have this aghori master acknowledge that you having this book in your hands now is a strong sign of divine blessings in your life, too.

Namaste.

About the Author

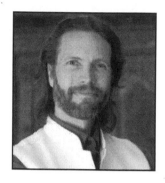

Dr. Clint G. Rogers, PhD is a university researcher who had no time for 'alternative medicine.' As a skeptic of anything outside the realm of Western science, he encountered the ancient healing world of Dr. Naram with a disposition ready to discount and minimize whatever he witnessed.

That was until modern medicine failed his own father, and Dr. Clint was left desperately searching for any solution to keep his father alive.

Through his TEDx talk, which has reached millions, and this new breakthrough book, *Ancient Secrets of a Master Healer,* Dr. Clint reveals how it was love for his father that pushed him beyond the barriers of what he thought was logical or possible, into a world in which 'healing miracles' are an everyday experience.

As of the publication of this book, Dr. Clint spent over 10 years traveling with Dr. Naram, documenting the ancient secrets, and helping more people know they exist.

In addition to this book and his TEDx talk, Dr. Clint designed and taught with Dr. Naram a university certification course in Berlin, Germany, for brilliant doctors from around the world, who wanted to learn and apply these ancient healing secrets.

Dr. Clint is currently the CEO of *Wisdom of the World Wellness*, an organization of dreamers and doers seeking out the best wisdom on the planet so everyone can benefit.

He is also a trustee of the *Ancient Secrets Foundation*, supporting humanitarian efforts which Dr. Naram loved.

Dr. Clint is passionate about sharing this form of deeper healing. Although not everyone may choose it, at least they should know that they have a choice.

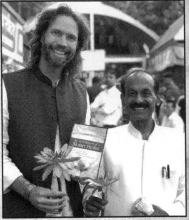

Printed in Poland
by Amazon Fulfillment
Poland Sp. z o.o., Wrocław